THE ULTIMATE STRESS BUSTER

THE ULTIMATE STRESS BUSTER

A seven-step plan for calm and relaxation

Dr Sarah Brewer

5 7 9 10 8 6 4

Text © Ebury Press 1999, 2003

Sarah Brewer has asserted her moral right to be identified as the author of this work in accordance with the Copyright, Design and Patents Act 1988.

First published in the United Kingdom in 1999 by Ebury

This edition published in 2003 by Vermilion, an imprint of Ebury Press

Random House UK Ltd.
Random House, 20 Vauxhall Bridge Road, London SW1V 2SA

Random House Australia (Pty) Limited
20 Alfred Street, Milsons Point, Sydney, New South Wales 2061, Australia

Random House New Zealand Limited
18 Poland Road, Glenfield, Auckland 10, New Zealand

Random House South Africa (Pty) Limited
Isle of Houghton, Corner of Boundary Road & Carse O'Gowrie,
Houghton 2198, South Africa

Random House UK Limited Reg. No. 954009

www.randomhouse.co.uk

Penguin Random House is committed to a sustainable future for our business, our readers and our planet. This book is made from Forest Stewardship Council® certified paper.

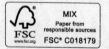

MIX
Paper from
responsible sources
FSC
www.fsc.org   FSC® C018179

Printed and bound in Great Britain by Clays Ltd, Elcograf S.p.A.
A CIP catalogue record is available for this book from the British Library.

ISBN: 9780091884512

CONTENTS

Introduction:

WHAT IS STRESS?

Stress is a modern term that simply means you are experiencing an abnormal amount of pressure. A certain amount of pressure is essential to help you meet life's challenges, release your creativity and fuel your continued personal growth. Once pressure falls outside the range with which you feel comfortable, however, it can lead to the unpleasant physical and emotional symptoms associated with distress.

Different people are comfortable with different amounts of pressure, and how you cope varies from person to person and even from time to time. One day you may feel totally calm and laid-back, able to cope with everything thrown your way, while on another occasion the slightest extra pressure will overwhelm you, turning you into a crumbling, tearful wreck. Sometimes you may even feel stressed because of insufficient pressure to drive your life forward. Being stuck in a boring rut with little stimulation can be just as frustrating and unpleasant as being loaded with too many tasks and not enough time. In some experiments performed in the 1950s, researchers put volunteers in a totally stress-free environment with no external stimulation of any kind. Within a short while some started to experience hallucinations and most felt disoriented – unsure of where they were and when. After three days, no amount of financial inducement could persuade the volunteers to continue staying in the totally stress-free, unstimulating environment.

Most musicians recognize that they perform better after feeling nervous before a concert starts, and Olympic athletes and professional actors normally need the presence of a live, interactive audience to achieve their full potential. When controlled, stress generates feelings of challenge, excitement and motivation. When uncontrolled, however, it produces extreme physical and emotional discomfort, bizarre behaviour, serious disease and ultimately premature death. It has been said that finding the right balance is like adjusting the strings of a musical instrument: too loose and the tune will be ruined; too tight and the strings will break. Just right, and the instrument will sing with a unique and lovely harmony that fills your mind, body and soul.

Why we feel stressed

Pressure is so important for survival that your body is programmed to produce a stress response known as the fight-or-flight reaction. It is this reaction – due mainly to the effects of adrenaline – that produces most of the physical and emotional feelings you experience when distressed. If your body did not produce adrenaline, feelings of stress would not occur, but as you would also not respond appropriately to the tasks and dangers of everyday life, you would not last long in the corporate and urban jungles of modern existence.

When you are confronted with a stressful situation, which may require increased physical activity, nerve signals from the brain trigger the release of adrenaline directly into your bloodstream. As a result, stress increases blood levels of adrenaline by as much as a thousandfold within just one minute. Adrenaline then produces an instant response in different parts of the body, so your whole system goes on to red alert.

- Your pulse rate, blood pressure and the force of your heart's contraction increase so more blood is pumped to your muscles and brain.

- Your circulation diverts blood away from the intestines towards your brain (for quick thinking), skeletal muscles (for exercise) and skin (for rapid cooling on exertion).

- Your sweat glands are switched on; you literally sweat with fear.

- Your muscles tense ready for action.

- Your breathing rate goes up and your airways widen to bring extra oxygen into your body.

- Your sugar levels increase as the body's stores are raised to provide instant energy for extra power, strength and speed.

- Your pupils dilate to improve your field of vision.

1st stage of stress reaction: Known as the fight-or-flight response – in which energy is mobilized within the body – this prepares the body for running away or for combat when you are under threat or pressure.

2nd stage of stress reaction: The effects of stress hormones would then be used up in vigorous exercise during fighting or fleeing which would soon neutralize the stress response and bring the body systems back into normal balance. Nowadays, the need to fight or flee rarely occurs so the effects of stress build up to make you jittery, taut and trembling inside.

3rd stage of stress reaction: This build-up of stress then develops into the third stage of the stress reaction – the potentially harmful stage – in which energy is drained from the body.

Other stress hormones

If stress continues for any length of time, the adrenal glands also increase their output of the steroid hormone, cortisol. This seems to be essential for survival, for if it does not occur (for example, if the adrenal glands are surgically removed) even slight stress may lead to sudden death unless steroid injections are given. Why this happens may be related to the fact that cortisol is needed to activate the rest of the sympathetic nervous system, helping to maintain blood pressure and to prevent the other physical effects of stress from becoming excessive. It may also be due to its role in releasing extra fatty acids into the circulation to act as an emergency energy supply. In the short term, this increase in cortisol levels is potentially life-saving. If stress continues, however, so cortisol levels remain persistently high, it can lead to harmful and disruptive symptoms. Any stimulus that increases secretion of cortisol from the adrenal cortex is described as a stressor (see Chapter 1).

Questionnaire

The body of a stressed person is affected both physically and mentally. Ask yourself these 12 questions to find out just how stressed you may be.

Yes No

1. Are you finding it difficult to concentrate and make simple decisions? ☐ ☐

2. Has your voice become more high-pitched and shrill, or do you suffer from a stiff jaw? ☐ ☐

3. Have you increased your intake of nicotine or alcohol? ☐ ☐

4. Are you over-breathing, which may show up as chest pains, tingling sensations, palpitations or asthma? ☐ ☐

5. Do you feel nauseous and suffer from ulcers, heartburn or indigestion? ☐ ☐

6. Do you sweat excessively or do you suffer from skin dryness or rashes? ☐ ☐

7. Is your immune system less efficient? ☐ ☐

8. Do you have difficulty in swallowing or does your mouth go dry? ☐ ☐

9. Does your neck ache, or do you suffer from backache, muscle tensions, fatigue or muscle pains? ☐ ☐

10. Do you have high blood pressure? Is your heart pumping faster or do you have palpitations? ☐ ☐

11. Do you suffer from tiredness, lethargy or sleep problems? ☐ ☐

12. Do you experience the need to urinate frequently, or suffer from diarrhoea? ☐ ☐

Your score: For each YES, score 1 point; for each NO, score 0 points.

1–3: You appear to be coping well with your everyday life and are not displaying any significant signs of stress.

4–9: You are showing some signs of stress. To help, make sure of Points 3–7 to reduce your stress levels before they get too great.

10–12: This signals an unduly high stress factor and you are advised to make large changes to your lifestyle to prevent illness.

Thinking positive

The power of mind over body should never be underestimated and is largely responsible for determining whether the adrenaline stress you experience has a positive or negative effect on your life.

When you think about it, there is obviously a vast difference between the enjoyable, anticipatory stress of excitement linked with positive thinking, and the worrying, down-dragging stress associated with negative emotions such as fear and anxiety. The same physical stress reactions are occurring in your body due to the release of adrenaline, but the way you respond to them is determined almost exclusively by your state of mind.

Imagine two people who have each been asked to give their first-ever speech to a large audience of over a hundred people at a work-related conference. Both face the same challenge, and experience the same stress reactions in their body – but one person feels in control, while the other feels terrified. The positive thinker looks on the task as a wonderful challenge, a chance to prove themselves at work, to gain experience in public speaking and to earn recognition and approval from those who are important for the advancement of their career. They picture the event in their mind and see themselves giving a flawless speech that holds the audience enthralled and impressed. The negative thinker, on the other hand, looks on the task with abject horror. Fear of failure, of getting muddled or tongue-tied and of making a fool of themselves takes over and they quake in their shoes, almost wishing they were dead. They picture the event in their mind and see themselves tripping up the steps, dropping their notes and fumbling their words. They just know they can't possibly do it properly and will end up being thought of as a complete idiot.

Both people experience the same stressful physical reactions in their body. The difference is how they mentally respond to them. The positive thinker responds to the high stress in a positive way and decides to prepare and practise thoroughly, so they will perform at their best. In contrast, the negative thinker responds to the high stress by becoming increasingly anxious, irritable and snappy. They feel trapped – there's no point in making any effort towards the coming disaster and no way to improve the outcome. They try to put the event from their mind and to survive through denial – perhaps they will even call in sick on the day.

When the big event arrives, both speakers feel the same nervous butterflies in their stomach, trembling hands, sweating and loose bowels. The positive thinker mentally rises to the challenge and copes brilliantly, however. Thanks to their careful preparation and the power of positive thought, they give an excellent speech that is well received. Afterwards, flushed with success, they bask in the glow of the limelight and can't wait to be asked to speak again. They have responded well to the positive stress and a new life skill has been learned.

The negative thinker experiences the humiliation of a self-fulfilling prophesy. They know they won't perform well, and they don't. They mumble their unpractised lines, fail to speak up so people can't hear at the back, and gabble through their talk too quickly, impressing no one – least of all themselves. The way they responded to the stress has adversely affected their performance and they have failed to cope. They have not learned a new skill and instead have learned to fear public speaking – the very thought of it will in future bring on a stress-related panic attack.

The way you think has a major effect on whether the stress you experience is beneficial or harmful. Some people are lucky and have learned a positive outlook on life from an early age. Others need to work hard to change the way they think. By thinking positive rather than negative thoughts, you can look on a stressful and difficult situation as a wonderful chance to learn new skills and acquire new experiences rather than seeing it through the fear of failure.

Try always to look for opportunities, not threats, as recent medical research suggests that negative emotions can be fatal. Over 300 men and women with heart disease were classed into negative thinkers (tendency to experience rather than express negative emotions) and non-negative thinkers. They were followed for ten years and it was found that the risk of premature death was nearly four times higher in those who had negative thoughts (27 per cent compared to 7 per cent). This effect was independent of other risk factors such as whether they also had high blood pressure or raised cholesterol levels and may well be related to the increased negative stress associated with negative thoughts. Inspector Dreyfus in *The Pink Panther* certainly had the right idea when he repeated his own positive personal mantra: 'Every day, in every way, I get better and better...' To help you think more positively, see Chapter 6.

Coping with stress

Although your stress response is largely automatic, you can consciously exert some control over two of its main features – your pattern of breathing and the amount of tension building up in your muscles.

When the body powers down from a high pressure situation, fight-or-flight is switched off and an opposite reaction is triggered called the rest-and-digest response. You can consciously help to switch off your stress response by altering your breathing pattern and by relaxing your muscles with a relaxation exercise. This starts to reverse some of the changes produced during the fight-or-flight reaction to stress so that digestion restarts, your breathing and heartbeat slow down and the tension in your muscles slowly recedes. To learn how to press your automatic reset button, see Chapter 5.

How you respond to stressful situations

Although it sounds like an obvious statement, it is worth emphasizing that whether or not you feel positive pressure or negative stress in a particular situation depends largely on the way you respond psychologically to that situation, or in other words, the way you interact with your environment. This is known as the 'interactional' model of stress, in which stress is thought to result from an imbalance between the demands being made on you (which may be real or perceived) and your ability (either real or perceived) to cope with them.

Whether or not you respond to the normal pressures of life in a stressed or non-stressed manner depends largely on your natural personality type, although you can learn how to change harmful behaviour traits.

Type A personalities: these people are more prone to experiencing high levels of stress and to have adverse effects as a result. They are easy to recognize as they are highly competitive, always setting tight deadlines for themselves and continually striving to get ahead, even in the little things of life. Type As usually look tense and distracted – often with hair awry from running their hands over their head. Despite the hype they generate about doing everything better than anyone else, Type A people are secretly quite insecure and need constant praise and reassurance.

Type B personalities: These personalities are self-assured, relaxed and pleasant to be with. They are equally motivated and get on with their tasks in an efficient, calm manner, using all the time they need. They wait patiently for attention, make excellent listeners and are rarely offensive. People with Type B personalities can achieve just as many goals as Type A and be just as ambitious, but the major difference is their lack of panic, aggression and stress while they do so. They are working to please themselves rather than others and therefore do not need to seek outside approval. As a result, they may sometimes seem quite unambitious, although this is not necessarily the case.

Type As tend to live to work, while Type Bs tend to work in order to live. They have many more outside interests and hobbies and therefore tend to be more interesting, well-rounded – and pleasant – people.

Type A personality traits

- Schedule more and more into less and less time.
- Constantly work against the clock, doing two things at once – often against real or imagined opposition from others.
- Deny feeling tired.
- Measure success in terms of numbers (for example, numbers of clients seen or items sold).
- Believe that if you want something done well you have to do it yourself.
- Become impatient watching others do things they feel they could do better or faster.
- Are obsessed with punctuality.
- Are angry, aggressive and impatient with delays and queues; hostile to anything or anyone getting in the way of their progress.
- Have difficulty coping with sitting down and doing nothing.
- Talk a lot, particularly about themselves and often in an explosive way.
- Swear a lot.
- Don't listen to other people's conversation or impatiently try to finish what others are saying for them.
- Make angry stabbing motions and other gesticulations with their hands.
- Click their tongue, nod their head, clench their fist, suck in air or pound the table when talking.
- Frequently jig their knee, drum their fingers or click their pen.
- Blink or lift their eyebrows rapidly.
- Fail to notice the beauty of things around them.
- Are very competitive and always play to win.

Type B personality traits

- Manage time and only book in what can reasonably be achieved in the time allowed.
- Never suffer from time urgency, and are therefore happy to do one thing at a time.
- Are able to work without agitation.
- Measure success in terms of quality of work and the pleasure derived from completing it properly.
- Delegate certain tasks to those more suited to them.
- Don't feel they have to impress others with their achievements unless the situation demands it.
- Feel pleased for others' success and tell them so.
- Are not bothered by lack of punctuality in themselves or others.
- Wait patiently in queues and adopt a philosophical approach to delays or mistakes.
- Don't have any free-floating hostility.
- Are happy to sit down and relax, doing nothing during quality time without guilt.
- Listen readily to others, giving them all the time they need to have their say.
- Rarely feel the need to swear.
- Tend to hold their body in a relaxed manner, with no obvious tension when talking.
- Readily appreciate the beauty of nature and art.
- Are pleasantly competitive – good losers who are always happy to see others win.

Which personality are you?

The distinction between Type A and Type B behaviour patterns is not clear cut, but forms a sliding scale. Most people recognize character traits from both personality types in themselves and are likely to fall somewhere between the two extremes. Answering these questions will help you determine whether you currently have a predominantly Type A, Type B or mixed personality. The word *currently* is important here, as it helps to underline the fact that you can learn new behaviour patterns, losing those that are harmful and gaining those that will help you to cope with excess pressure.

Score each of the following questions as: Always = 5, Usually = 4, Sometimes = 3, Rarely = 2, Never = 1

☐ Are you ambitious?

☐ Do you always play to win and hate to lose?

☐ Are you on-the-dot punctual and hate being late?

☐ Are you eager to get things done as quickly as possible?

☐ Do you feel rushed?

☐ Do you get aggressive if frustrated?

☐ Are you impatient and angry when kept waiting?

☐ Do you tend to anticipate what others are going to say and finish their sentence for them?

❑ Do you interrupt others rather than waiting for them to have their say?

❑ Do you try to do too many things at once?

❑ Do you think ahead to the next things you have to do?

❑ Do you speak in a rapid, forceful manner?

❑ Do you eat or walk quickly?

❑ Do you gesticulate when you talk?

❑ Do you jiggle your knee, tap your fingers, click your pen or have to have something on the go rather than sitting quietly and relaxing?

❑ Are you a slave-driver who pushes yourself and others too hard?

❑ Do you want a good job, well done by yourself, to be recognized as such by others?

❑ Do you hide or suppress your feelings?

❑ Does your whole life revolve around work and home, with few hobbies or outside interests?

❑ Do you feel you have to do everything yourself and find it hard to delegate to others?

SCORE OVER 80: Driven Type A

You always put more pressure on yourself than necessary in your striving for success. In the long term, this will contribute to high stress levels and increase your risk of ill health if you don't take steps to change your behaviour patterns.

SCORE 65–80: Moderate Type A
You are a moderate Type A and need to watch that in striving for success, you do not push yourself too far. Ease back a little and make things easier on yourself. Take more time out for relaxation, and try to keep in touch with your inner self.

SCORE 56–64: Mixed Type A/Type B
Your personality displays a combination of Type A and Type B behaviour. You potentially have the best of both behavioural traits but need to ensure the Type A behaviour does not start to dominate as your ambitions grow. Continue to let pressure wash over you as much as possible so that it does not lead to physical or emotional symptoms of stress.

SCORE 40–55: Towards Type B
You have a healthy approach to life and are likely to achieve great things without harmful levels of stress. You are unlikely to suffer from stress-related illnesses.

SCORE BELOW 40: Laid-back Type B
You have a totally laid-back approach to life and are rarely stressed by very much. You need to keep you eyes on your life's goals to ensure you achieve them in your allotted time-span. Assuming you are sufficiently ambitious, you can achieve great things without panic and are unlikely to succumb to stress-related illnesses.

Ways of reducing Type A behaviour

If you recognize you have Type A characteristics, try to become aware of the effect your behaviour has on others, who may see you as overly hostile. A number of strategies, detailed later in this book, will help you learn to move away from Type A behaviour so you become more of a Type B personality. It is also helpful to select a Type B friend and adapt your own excessive behaviour traits to match their less aggressive approach to life. Or you can use the structured steps listed below. These changes should be made slowly over a period of time until they became part of your normal behaviour pattern: don't attempt to assimilate them quickly in your usual harassed manner.

1: Realign your priorities and aim for things worth being rather than things worth having.

2: Aim to stop being an idealist or perfectionist – accept that things can go wrong without it necessarily being the fault of yourself or others. Don't automatically look for someone to blame.

3: Don't keep looking for excuses to be disappointed – start looking for excuses to say 'well done' or 'thank you' to others.

4: Try being more relaxed and positive. Realize that Type B personalities may be just as ambitious as Type As, but they manage to reach their goals without seeming to panic.

5: Force yourself to listen to what others have to say – and let them finish their sentences. Rather than butting in, stop and ask yourself whether you really have anything important to say, whether anyone would want to hear it, and if so whether this is the time to say it.

6: Learn to laugh at yourself rather than at other people.

7: Learn to prioritize your tasks by making a 'To Do' list and seeing what can wait until tomorrow rather than having to be done today.

8: Learn to delegate appropriate tasks, even if you think you can do the job better alone.

9: Make decisions in unhurried circumstances – they are more likely to be good decisions than those made in haste.

10: Don't make unnecessary appointments or meetings.

11: Learn to be patient. Try talking more slowly, and practise waiting in a queue without getting frustrated.

12: Take regular 'time-out' breaks during your day where you relax.

13: Put aside one evening a week for personal pleasure – to visit the theatre, for example, or read a good book while listening to a relaxation tape.

14: Start taking regular non-competitive exercise to reduce your levels of stress – brisk walking, gentle jogging, swimming or cycling are ideal. Avoid squash.

15: Stop watching the clock: try not wearing a watch and taking the clock off the wall.

16: Practise telling people how you feel: talk about your emotions rather than bottling them up.

Learning to cope

The key to successful stress management is to obtain the right balance between pressures you can handle and the overload that drags you down. In this respect, the crucial balance is not usually that between demands on you and your actual capability, but between the way you perceive these demands in relation to how you think you can cope.

Coping with stress is not a lucky trait some people are born with and others not – it is a skill that can be learned and perfected, just like any other in life. Those who cope best with stress are those who see challenges as a normal, positive part of life; who feel in control, are committed to their work, hobbies, social life or family, and who see challenges as opportunities rather than threats.

The fact that you are prepared to make changes in your behaviour shows that you are willing to adapt to help cope with the excess stress you are experiencing. Adaptation is vital to survive and cope with longer term stress. There are two ways of adapting, however, and one is successful, the other not. It is therefore important to make sure the adaptive moves you make are going to work, which means not becoming clouded by unhelpful defence mechanisms.

These are subconscious ways of distorting reality and are rarely helpful in coping with prolonged or excessive stress. These include:

- The well-known ostrich-head-in-the-sand approach: pretend it isn't there and it will go away. While this can be helpful for short periods of time, it becomes counter-productive if it persists and you start distorting reality in different ways to maintain the fiction. The source of stress rarely goes away, and even if it seems to, the anxiety that it will return continues to lurk and provoke feelings of inadequacy and doom.

- Always blame everyone else when things go wrong – by projecting the problem on to others, you automatically lose the need to feel responsible yourself.
- Rationalize everything away and to find acceptable excuses for things that really are quite unacceptable.
- You may also try to cope by isolating problems and talking about them in a cold, clinical and unfeeling way.

The only defence mechanism that has a chance of being successful is sublimation – the substitution of acceptable for unacceptable activity (for example, channelling aggression into playing sport). However, if the sport involved is a competitive one, then stress levels may not improve as a result of increased physical activity, as the pressure to win may overwhelm any enjoyment that might be obtained from participating.

In place of unhelpful defence mechanisms look for adaptive coping mechanisms, which are explained in detail in Chapters 3 to 7. These are deliberate ways of adjusting to stress in a positive and constructive manner. They include recognizing when you are experiencing negative stress, developing self-esteem, eating wisely, taking exercise, relaxing, exploring alternative therapies and streamlining your life

How stressed are you?

It is hard to be objective about your own levels of stress as they can vary from day to day and week to week. The key is how well you are coping with your current stress levels and their effects on your quality of life. Answer these questions to work out your level of stress.

Score the following questions: A (not at all), B (sometimes, but not enough to be a major problem) or C (yes, very much so)

☐ Do you worry about your physical health?

☐ Do you worry about your emotional health?

☐ Do you worry about the future?

☐ Are you under financial strain?

☐ Is your motivation failing?

☐ Does your workload seem heavy?

☐ Do you feel uncomfortable with your job?

☐ Do you feel your work colleagues could be more supportive?

☐ Do you feel exhausted at the end of the day?

☐ Are you late for work?

☐ Have you been off sick from work?

☐ Do you feel uncomfortable with your social life?

☐ Do you worry about the amount of alcohol you are drinking or feel you ought to cut back?

☐ Do you feel your family and friends could be more supportive?

☐ If you smoke, has your need to do so increased?

☐ Are you sleeping badly?

☐ Do you get irritable or lose your temper?

☐ Do you feel trapped with no way to escape?

☐ Are you so busy you do not have time to relax?

☐ Do you wish you could drop everything and escape to a desert island?

INTERPRETATION

MOSTLY As: You are so laid-back that life seems too perfect for words. Either life is passing you by with few challenges and little room for personal growth, or there are very few goals left that you want to achieve. Re-evaluate where you are in comparison to where you want to be and assess whether a little more pressure might actually be beneficial. If not, then congratulations. You probably do not need to continue reading this book!

MOSTLY Bs: You are in the lucky situation of having achieved a balance between the challenges in your life and your ability to cope. Stress is not a major problem for you – yet – but you need to keep it that way. The following chapters will help you maintain your equilibrium in life.

MOSTLY Cs: You are under excess pressure and if this continues, stress will affect your health if it hasn't already done so. You cannot go on like this. It is imperative that you take a well-earned break and closely follow the advice given in the rest of this book. It is time to make significant changes to your work and lifestyle – or by the time you have achieved your ambitions in life you may no longer be fit to reap the benefits.

1 SPOT THE SIGNS OF STRESS

Excess stress affects different people in different ways at different times in their life. Your ability to cope will depend on several factors, such as your overall health, whether you are personality Type A or B, whether you tend to think positive or negative thoughts, the way you've learned to cope in the past and the number of stressful events you have recently experienced, one after the other, without sufficient time to recover in between. Your overall health is particularly important because if you are already experiencing physical or emotional stress due to the symptoms of another illness, your reserves of coping will already be partly used up. Even a little additional external stress may mean you are unable to cope any more. Women also have the additional disadvantage that their menstrual cycle can cause symptoms of internal stress regularly each month (see page 121), and in middle age around the time of the menopause (see page 117). If you are anxious about change, have poor self-esteem or feel you are losing control of a situation, this will automatically make your symptoms of stress seem worse.

By learning how to spot the signs of stress, you are more able to take steps to reduce the pressure you are under before stress sets in long-term and your physical or emotional health starts to suffer. Stress affects different people in different ways. Some are more likely to develop physical distress, some experience serious psychological or emotional problems while others show worrying behavioural changes. It is useful to consider the symptoms of stress in the following categories, which broadly represent increasingly severe reactions:

- **Level 1:** Early warning signs
- **Level 2:** Psychological symptoms
- **Level 3:** Emotional symptoms
- **Level 4:** Physical symptoms
- **Level 5:** Behavioural symptoms
- **Level 6:** Breakdown

You can experience symptoms from different levels of stress at the same time. These levels tend to represent a natural gradation, however. Those under less stress are likely to experience more of the psychological and emotional symptoms, while those under greater levels of stress are likely to experience more of the physical symptoms. By the time you reach the stage of breakdown (which hopefully you never will) you might experience most of the symptoms associated with each level of stress all at the same time.

Level 1: Early warning signs

When you feel stressed, you are usually aware of excess pressure and may describe yourself as being (tick the ones that apply to you):

- [ ] uneasy
- [ ] on edge
- [ ] tense
- [ ] hassled
- [ ] flustered
- [ ] uptight

- [ ] under pressure
- [ ] taut
- [ ] overloaded
- [ ] about to explode
- [ ] without your sense of humour
- [ ] at the end of your tether

Everyone will have experienced these early warning signs at some time. You may notice that you are becoming clumsy or restless, pacing up and down, fiddling with jewellery or – men especially – jingling coins in your trouser pocket. Your speech may be affected, so you find yourself hesitating, speaking too fast, too quietly/loudly or even stammering and stuttering. You may also find yourself putting things off – avoiding facing issues that may prove difficult. Most of all, however, you will probably notice strong emotional feelings such as irritability, anger, impatience and that you are constantly looking for – and finding – faults in others. You are likely to start feeling tired and irritable, to develop tension headaches and to notice some disturbance of your normal sleep patterns.

Quick tips to stop stress in its tracks

- Stop what you are doing and inwardly say, 'Calm!' to yourself.

- If you are sitting down, stand up and gently stretch to your fullest possible extent.

- Take a deep breath in and let it out slowly, concentrating on the movement of your diaphragm. Do this two or three times until you start to feel more in control. (See also breathing in Chapter 4.)

- Shake your hands and arms briskly, then shrug your shoulders.

- If possible, go for a brisk walk, even if it is only briefly around the room or to the bathroom, to help get your circulation going again.

- If possible, go somewhere private and groan or shout as loudly as you can. This can be very therapeutic. Some people find it helpful to punch a soft cushion as hard as possible.

- Place a few drops of Bach Flower Rescue Remedy on your tongue.

- Inhale a personally chosen blend of aromatherapy oils made by adding a total of 15 drops of essential oils to 30 ml of carrier oil (e.g. almond and grapeseed oil). Select two or three oils to blend from the following: bergamot, cardamom, camomile, coriander, geranium, grapefruit, lavender, lemon, neroli, sandalwood.

- Choose an appropriate, personal positive thought (for example, 'I am feeling positive pressure, not negative stress') and repeat this regularly to yourself during a visualization exercise (see page 193).

Level 2: Psychological symptoms

Prolonged stress leads to depletion of mental as well as physical energy and can result in a number of psychological symptoms that in turn reduce your ability to cope with the original problem. When you start to experience the psychological symptoms of stress, you know that your ability to cope is under threat. At this stage it is important to practise the 'Quick tips' given on page 31 and to start introducing more long-term stress-coping strategies. Place a tick next to any of the following psychological symptoms of stress from which you frequently suffer.

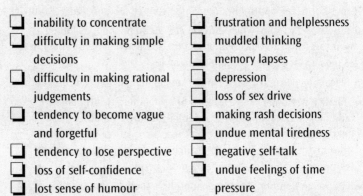

- ☐ inability to concentrate
- ☐ difficulty in making simple decisions
- ☐ difficulty in making rational judgements
- ☐ tendency to become vague and forgetful
- ☐ tendency to lose perspective
- ☐ loss of self-confidence
- ☐ lost sense of humour
- ☐ frustration and helplessness
- ☐ muddled thinking
- ☐ memory lapses
- ☐ depression
- ☐ loss of sex drive
- ☐ making rash decisions
- ☐ undue mental tiredness
- ☐ negative self-talk
- ☐ undue feelings of time pressure

If you ticked three or more symptoms, you are likely to be experiencing a significant amount of psychological stress.

Attack plan to help reduce your stress levels

- Make sure you are eating a healthy diet and that you do not skip meals. Have healthy snacks to hand such as dried or fresh fruit, rice cakes or oatcakes to help stop your blood sugar levels from falling and creating an additional internal trigger for the negative stress response.

- If you are not taking regular exercise, now is the time to start (see Chapter 4).

- Learn a breathing/relaxation technique to use when your mind starts to feel like cotton wool (see Chapter 4).

- Cut back on any excesses such as alcohol intake, cigarette-smoking or reliance on recreational drugs.

- If practical, try listening to calming background music to help you unwind.

- Start learning assertiveness techniques – saying no to unreasonable demands helps to reduce the pressure you are under (see Chapter 6).

- Start organizing your life and managing your time more effectively (see Chapter 7).

- Award yourself a special weekly treat (for example, an aromatherapy massage) as a reward for coping and for being such a wonderful person.

- Make a point of complementing others around you – if you make them feel good about themselves, the effects will wear off on you too.

Level 3: Emotional symptoms

When you experience emotional symptoms of stress, your ability to cope is under threat of being overwhelmed and your energy reserves approach depletion. You may already have started to experience some of the physical symptoms of stress (see page 36) and if you do not take steps to reduce the amount of negative stress you are under, this will start to take a toll on your health. Continue practising your Level 1 and 2 strategies and introduce more advanced strategies to help you reduce the tension you are under. Place a tick next to any of the following emotional symptoms of stress from which you frequently suffer:

- [ ] overwhelming feelings of anxiety
- [ ] angry outbursts
- [ ] feeling isolated
- [ ] defensive and over-sensitive to criticism
- [ ] fear of failure
- [ ] feelings of guilt
- [ ] resentment or animosity

- [ ] feeling of depression
- [ ] irritability
- [ ] feeling of hopelessness
- [ ] increased cynicism
- [ ] fear of rejection
- [ ] nightmares
- [ ] feeling of hostility
- [ ] undue aggression
- [ ] panic attacks

If you ticked three or more boxes, you are likely to be experiencing a significant amount of emotional stress.

Attack plan to reduce your stress levels further

- Work out what situations or people are causing you stress and why, then see if you can formulate sensible strategies to overcome the problem.

- Keep a stress diary (see page 132).

- Learn how to prioritize tasks so you can deal with pressures one at a time.

- Practise positive thinking techniques or visualization to help boost your flagging self-confidence.

- Develop more hobbies and interests to help you relax and take your mind off your worries.

- Watch a favourite comedy film, comedian or humorous play and try to laugh as much as possible – laughter is a wonderful antidote to building stress. Similarly, if you feel like a good cry, then have one and get it out of your system. We are the only animals who cry, and shedding tears does seem to act as an emergency reset button to help relieve excess tension.

- Treat yourself to an extra aromatherapy massage, facial or other body treatment to make you feel better in yourself.

- Consider enrolling in a yoga or t'ai chi class.

- Use visualization to help you achieve a more relaxed state of mind.

- Consider having a few days' holiday relaxing at home so you can recharge your internal batteries.

Level 4: Physical symptoms

If you have persistent physical symptoms, you have excess adrenaline and other stress hormones circulating in your bloodstream. Long-term high levels of stress dampen your immunity and are linked with an increased risk of a number of important illnesses, including coronary heart disease and possibly even some cancers. Place a tick next to any of the following symptoms that are persistent:

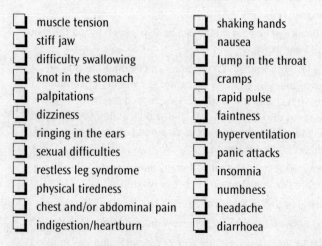

- muscle tension
- stiff jaw
- difficulty swallowing
- knot in the stomach
- palpitations
- dizziness
- ringing in the ears
- sexual difficulties
- restless leg syndrome
- physical tiredness
- chest and/or abdominal pain
- indigestion/heartburn
- shaking hands
- nausea
- lump in the throat
- cramps
- rapid pulse
- faintness
- hyperventilation
- panic attacks
- insomnia
- numbness
- headache
- diarrhoea

If you ticked three or more symptoms, you are likely to be experiencing a significant amount of physical stress.

Advanced plan to reduce high stress levels

- Review your stress diary regularly to help identify your main causes of stress so you can formulate sensible plans to overcome them.

- Consider having a few days' holiday at home.

- Learn how to meditate so you can find an inner spot of calm when all around you is in a state of tension or chaos (see page 188).

- Surround yourself with calming colours.

- Take special care to eat a healthy, wholefood, organic diet.

- Take a good vitamin and mineral supplement providing around 100 per cent of as many vitamins and minerals as possible. You may need extra B-group vitamins if you are feeling tired all the time.

- Take an additional antioxidant supplement so you are obtaining at least:

  - 500–1,000 mg vitamin C per day (ester-C is best as it is non-acidic – check labels to find it)

  - 400 IU vitamin E daily.

- Consider taking coenzyme Q10 to help boost oxygen usage by your cells and to improve your energy levels.

- Take evening primrose oil (at least 1,000 mg daily) to help correct any hormone imbalances resulting from increased stress.

- Consider taking an adaptogenic herb such as American, Korean or Siberian ginseng (see pages 148–150). Take ginseng for six weeks initially, then continue on a two weeks on, two weeks off cycle.

Level 5: Behavioural symptoms

Someone under severe stress will make changes in their behaviour in an attempt to avoid or mask their problems. These changes are often subconscious and are easily recognizable as a sign that they need urgent help. Although in many ways behavioural symptoms represent a self-protective mechanism, they never solve the problem and soon become a source of additional stress in their own right. The fact that your stress levels are linked with behavioural changes should sound a loud warning bell. You need to reduce your levels of stress NOW because they lead to a total inability to cope – a condition commonly described as a nervous breakdown. Continue practising your Level 1, 2, 3 and 4 coping strategies and also take steps to address the behavioural changes you have adopted.

Place a tick next to any of the following behavioural symptoms of stress from which you frequently suffer:

- ☐ avoidance of certain people and places
- ☐ social withdrawal
- ☐ phobic avoidance of certain situations or things
- ☐ absenteeism
- ☐ becoming a workaholic with no time for relaxation
- ☐ hair-pulling
- ☐ increased reliance on alcohol and/or cigarettes and/or tranquillizers

☐ changes in eating patterns: increased or decreased food intake that affects body weight

☐ obsessive or compulsive behaviour, for example frequent hand-washing, checking and re-checking you have switched off lights or locked doors

If you ticked three or more symptoms you are likely to be displaying significant behavioural symptoms of stress.

Attack plan to help reduce your behavioural symptoms of stress

- Make plans to cut back on your alcohol intake (see page 76).

- Take steps to cut back on the number of cigarettes you smoke. Once you feel stronger you can attempt to stop altogether (see page 91).

- Seek help to rethink unhealthy behaviour patterns and learn new ones – hypnotherapy may be helpful (see page 184).

- Cut back on your working hours and build regular rest or exercise breaks into your day. Make a point of doing at least one activity you enjoy for at least 30 minutes each day and preferably longer.

- Arrange to have a therapeutic massage at least once a week.

- Address absenteeism by taking a planned holiday (preferably at home) then starting back at work with a promise to yourself that you will continue going in, no matter what. If problems at work need addressing, raise issues with the appropriate manager.

The signs of stress

There are a great number of symptoms that can signal stress, ranging from feeling tired all the time and great feelings of anger to insomnia and indigestion and heartburn. The following pages form a reference guide to the main symptoms that might indicate you are suffering from undue levels to stress:

Alopecia (page 41)
Anger (page 42)
Anxiety and panic attacks
  (page 44)
Asthma (page 48)
Chest pain (page 50)
Cramp (page 51)
Depression (page 53)
Eczema (page 56)
Hair-pulling (page 58)
Headaches and migraine
  (page 60)
High blood pressure (page 62)
Impotence (page 65)

Indigestion and heartburn
  (page 66)
Infections (page 68)
Insomnia (page 70)
Irritability (page 74)
Irritable bowel syndrome
  (page 78)
Memory (page 81)
Phobias (page 83)
Psoriasis (page 85)
Restless legs syndrome (page 87)
Sex drive (page 88)
Tired all the Time (TATT) (page 93)
TMJ syndrome (page 95)

Alopecia

Alopecia is a common hair loss condition that can be linked with stress. It occurs when certain hair follicles stop growing, either in a small patch of skin, on one region of the body or occasionally all over the body. The cause of alopecia seems to be related to abnormal activity of the immune system, which attacks or switches off certain hair follicles. Stress plays a major role because stress can affect immune function and because it leads to tightness of the scalp plus contraction of blood vessels in the area, which reduces blood supply to the hair follicles.

Self-help

- Massage your scalp with your fingers for five to ten minutes per day to boost circulation.

- Lift handfuls of hair and use these to gently push and pull your scalp over the underlying bone to help loosen any tense tissues.

- Take Bach Flower Rescue Remedy drops whenever you feel stressed; massage Rescue Remedy Cream into the bald areas of scalp.

- Aromatherapy: Massage the bare patch twice a week with essential oils of rosemary and lavender diluted with almond or jojoba oil, see page 173. (Do not use aromatherapy if pregnant or if you have high blood pressure or epilepsy without seeking advice, see page 174.)

- Occasionally alopecia is linked with lack of iron or an underactive thyroid – ask your doctor if you need blood tests.

Anger

Anger is a potentially destructive emotion that results when stress and frustration build up beyond your ability to cope. Anger uses up a lot of energy and triggers a high level of internal emotional and physical stress, which stops you thinking rationally. Anger often results when:

- You feel frustrated at not being able to do what you want, when you want.
- You can't get your own way.
- People do not do what you expect them to do.
- You cannot find the words to express yourself properly.
- Communication breaks down.

Some people bottle up their anger, others let it out. All forms of anger are stressful and unhealthy.

Self-help

- Anger comes from your thoughts, and learning to think in a different way is an effective method of defusing your anger response.
- It also helps to become more assertive – so you are not put upon – and to learn how to express your emotions more fully. By allowing someone else to make you feel angry, you are giving them power over you. To remove this power, you need to take responsibility for your own anger and realize that you are in control of it, nobody else.

To help yourself do this, use 'I' language – 'I am angry because...' rather than 'You/They/This makes me angry because...'.

- Keep an anger diary to record exactly when you feel angry and why. If you can work out the triggers that arouse your emotions, you can help to circumvent them at an early stage.

- Try to delay your anger rather than acting immediately as this starts letting you feel in control of it. If possible, try to reduce its level, so you let yourself feel dismayed or disappointed rather than angry.

- Accept that you do not have a right to expect other people or things to be exactly how you want them to be – we live in an imperfect world and therefore need to be flexible and accept compromise.

- When you feel anger rising, practise a slow breathing exercise and consciously try to relax. This is your personal equivalent of biting your tongue or counting to ten.

- Use an appropriate personal affirmation such as, 'I will not feel angry, I will stay in control' or, 'Keep cool, calm and collected', and keep repeating this to yourself when appropriate.

- If you are too angry to think straight, then say 'I'll discuss this later' and move away from the situation temporarily. When you feel in control again, go back and address the issue – don't avoid it.

- When you are on your own, pretend the person or situation that made you feel angry is present and describe out loud exactly how you feel. Say all the things you want to say to that person or in that situation, to get them out of your system.

Anxiety and panic attacks

Anxiety is one of the main symptoms of stress and is associated with feelings of apprehension, dread, panic and impending doom. While short-lived anxiety is appropriate in some situations (for example, when going for an interview), those with morbid anxiety worry excessively about trivial matters and frequently experience other typical stress symptoms such as restlessness, palpitations, tremor, flushing, dizziness, hyperventilation, loose bowels, sweating, muscle tension and insomnia.

Anxiety often results from internal sources of stress and typically develops between the late teens and early thirties when it may also be associated with excess intakes of caffeine, alcohol or illegal drugs. Anxiety occurring later in life may be part of a depressive illness. In eight out of ten cases, anxiety due to internal stress is self-limiting and resolves within a few weeks following reassurance and emotional support such as counselling, behaviour therapy or relaxation techniques. In some cases, however, anxiety becomes worse and may develop into panic attacks.

Panic attacks are surprisingly common – an estimated one in 20 people suffer on a regular basis. Many of those who suffer can remember the exact occasion when they experienced their first attack, such as in a crowded supermarket or following a series of stressful events at work. If you suffer from panic attacks but cannot remember any particular trigger, some psychologists believe your fear may date from an event in early childhood which is stored in your subconscious memory.

Over-breathing

Panic attacks are now thought to be triggered by over-breathing – a condition known as hyperventilation syndrome. During times of extreme stress, your breathing pattern changes as part of the fight-or-flight response, so you take quick, irregular, shallow breaths that help to draw in more oxygen more quickly. This in turn means you blow off more carbon dioxide – a waste acid gas produced by your metabolism. If you continue hyperventilating, you will soon exhale so much carbon dioxide that your blood loses acidity and becomes increasingly alkaline. This affects the transmission of nerve signals and causes physical symptoms of dizziness, faintness and pins and needles. These symptoms heighten your sense of panic so you tend to breathe even faster, blowing off even more carbon dioxide, to trigger a panic attack.

People who habitually hyperventilate sometimes experience frightening physical symptoms, including chest pain, palpitations, visual disturbances, numbness, severe headache, insomnia and even collapse. It is important to seek medical advice if these occur – don't make the diagnosis of panic attack yourself or it is possible that a more serious problem (for example, a heart condition) may be missed.

Many people under stress feel as if they have a lump in their throat and develop difficulty in swallowing. It used to be thought that this was due to abnormal muscle contraction in the oesophagus but researchers have now found this sensation can be brought on in most people just by over-breathing.

Self-help

- Concentrate on breathing slowly, deeply and quietly to prevent hyperventiliation.

- When you feel panic rising say, 'Stop it!' quietly to yourself and breathe in and out slowly.

- If panic continues to rise, cup your hands over your nose and mouth so you breathe back some of the excess carbon dioxide gas you have blown off.

- If you are somewhere private, breathe in and out of a paper bag.

- Don't escalate the panic by worrying about what is going to happen.

- Try to distract your thoughts by studying your surroundings as you wait for the attack to pass – symptoms usually subside quickly.

- Stay in the situation if practical and you are in no physical danger. If you run away rather than facing your fear, it will be more difficult to cope and to avoid another panic attack when you experience the same situation again.

- Talk to someone about your worries, either a valued friend or a professional counsellor, to help off-load your feelings so they don't build up inside. And if you are going somewhere or doing something stressful that has previously caused a panic attack, ask a trusted, sympathetic person such as a close friend or relative to go with you for moral support.

- If your symptoms are debilitating, you may benefit from anxiety management training with a behaviour therapist. You will be taught how to reduce your anxiety through relaxation, distraction and reassuring affirmations such as, 'I can cope'. If panic attacks are becoming troublesome, ask your GP for advice about joining a therapy group or receiving individual psychotherapy.

- Take regular exercise such as swimming, walking or cycling to help burn off stress hormones.

- Avoid excessive caffeine.

- Take a good multinutrient supplement containing as many vitamins and minerals as possible at around 100 per cent of the recommended daily amount (RDA).

- Eat little and often to keep your blood sugar levels up – never skip a meal, especially breakfast.

- Cut back on sugar, salt, saturated fats and convenience foods.

- Watch your alcohol intake and try to limit yourself to a maximum of one or two alcoholic drinks per day.

- Look into alternative therapies such as acupressure, Bach Flower remedies, herbalism, hypnotherapy, reflexology and visualization (see Chapter 5).

Asthma

Asthma is a long-term inflammatory disease of the lungs. The number of sufferers has doubled over the last 30 years and it is now especially common in women of all ages – two out of three sufferers are female. The reasons for this are unknown, but one theory is that women are now under more stress from having to juggle work and family pressures.

When asthma is triggered, the airways go into spasm. This produces the symptoms of coughing, wheezing, tightness in the chest and shortness of breath. The other signs of inflammation – swelling and extra mucus secretion – take longer to come on and often result in a further bout of tightness and wheezing 6–8 hours later. In severe cases, airway narrowing and plugs of mucus can block the flow of oxygen into the lungs.

Symptoms occur when the lining of the airways becomes red and swollen and produces increased amounts of mucus. Once irritation sets in, the airways become increasingly sensitive to a range of triggers such as exercise, strong emotions – including stress – and air-borne particles.

Self-help

- Eating more fish may be beneficial – aim for 100 g oily fish two or three times per week, or try omega-3 fish oil supplements.
- Asthma has also been linked with low dietary levels of selenium, magnesium or B6 in some studies, while those with high intakes of antioxidants (vitamin E or vitamin C) seemed to have the lowest risk.

- If you think you have stress-related asthma, you should be assessed regularly by your doctor so that adequate treatment is given.
- Stop smoking – and try to avoid smoky places.
- Wear a special mask when exercising near traffic.
- Keep the home as dust-free as possible. Dusting with a damp cloth and using a vacuum cleaner with a special filter will help. A spray that kills off dust mites is available from chemists. Spray on to beds, curtains and carpets every three months.
- Put special covers over your mattress, pillow and duvet to overcome bedmites.
- If you have asthma, avoid taking aspirin or ibuprofen, which can trigger an attack.
- Take your medication correctly, as prescribed.
- Ask the practice nurse or doctor to check your inhaler technique is good.

Chest pain

Severe stress can lead to chest pain, which may be due to spasm of muscles in the chest wall or, more seriously, to spasm of the coronary arteries supplying blood and oxygen to the heart. This triggers heart muscle pain (angina) which is usually felt behind the chest bone, is described as tight and crushing – like a bear hug or as spreading through the chest and may radiate up into the neck, jaw or down the left arm. Angina may also be brought on by exertion and relieved by rest if circulation to the heart is impaired by hardening and furring up of the arteries.

If heart muscle cells die due to prolonged oxygen starvation, a heart attack occurs. Heart attack pain is similar to angina but it lasts longer, is more intense, is usually accompanied by sweating, paleness and breathlessness and can come on at any time and is unrelieved by rest. Sudden chest pain should always be taken seriously and medical assistance sought.

Self-help

- Stop smoking and you will reduce the rick of coronary heart disease by 50–70 per cent within five years.

- Exercise regularly and the risk will be at 45 per cent lower.

- By losing excess weight the risk will be at 35–55 per cent lower.

- Stick to 2–3 units of alcohol/day and the risk will be at 25–45 per cent lower.

Cramp

Cramp is the popular name for a painful, excessive contraction of a muscle. This is usually felt in the leg, but any muscle can be affected. Cramps are linked with a build-up of lactic acid and other waste products of muscle metabolism – usually during or after physical exercise. They can also occur when you are stressed, however, and your muscles are held unusually tense for prolonged periods of time. When stressed and working long hours, cramps can also be related to sitting in an awkward position for too long.

Self-help

- Cramps can usually be relieved by vigorous massage, applying a hot or cold compress, or by gently stretching the affected muscle.

- Recurrent night cramps can often be relieved by taking supplements of calcium or quinine and by ensuring you drink enough fluids during the day.

- Increase your dietary intake of calcium (for example, low-fat milk, cheese, yoghurt, dark-green leafy vegetables) and magnesium (nuts, seafood, dairy products, wholegrains, dark green leafy vegetables).

- Improve a poor circulation with garlic tablets, ginkgo extracts and omega-3 fish-oil supplements.

- Consider taking coenzyme Q10, which increases oxygen uptake in muscle cells, especially when circulation is poor.

- Rub St John's wort oil or eucalyptus oil into the affected muscle to dilate small blood vessels and help relax tense muscle fibres.

- Some nutritionists suggest combining one tablespoon of apple cider vinegar and one tablespoon of honey in a glass and drinking daily.

- Add five drops of rosemary essential oil to a warm bath and relax before going to bed.

- Warm up and stretch for at least 15 minutes before starting exercise.

- Start exercising slowly and gradually build up your exertion.

- Take a good vitamin and mineral supplement that includes calcium, magnesium and vitamin E.

- Try taking the homeopathic remedy, Cuprum metallicum 6c.

Depression

Few people are blessed with a happy mood all the time. One day you may feel cheerful, energetic and lively, while the next you feel gloomy, listless and withdrawn, especially if you are under pressure. These mood swings are a normal part of everyday life, but sometimes they can get out of hand and if your mood swings too low, mild depression can occur.

Depression is often associated with long-term periods of excess pressure, and as many as one in eight men and one in five women will suffer from severe depression at some time during their life. It is one of the most common reasons why people consult their doctor, yet it is estimated that only half of all cases are diagnosed, since many sufferers either do not realize they have a depressive illness or are unwilling to seek help. This is especially likely in those under severe stress who may perceive emotional symptoms as a sign of weakness.

Depression is caused by an imbalance of the chemical messengers in the brain that are responsible for passing signals from one brain cell to another. If levels of one or more of these fall too low, the brain does not function properly and a variety of psychological and physical symptoms can occur including:

- A general slowing down
- Nervousness, anxiety and agitation
- Constant feelings of tiredness or exhaustion
- Headache

- Difficulty concentrating
- Loss of self-esteem and lack of confidence
- Preoccupation with your health
- Low sex drive
- Loss of interest in life
- Low mood with crying and sadness
- Loss of interest in everyday life

These symptoms are similar to those occurring during times of extreme stress, and the two conditions are often linked. With more severe depression, symptoms such as poor appetite, weight loss, difficulty sleeping and early morning waking (typically around 3am) develop.

Mild depression may eventually get better on its own, but your mood may dip even lower until you are suffering from a full-blown depressive illness. People suffering from moderate to severe depression are unlikely to snap out of their low mood without treatment with counselling and/or antidepressant therapy. If you think you are depressed, it is important to consult your doctor.

Self-help

- Make a 'To Do' list of a few simple tasks to achieve each day, even when you don't feel like doing much at all.
- Take care of your personal appearance – even though there may

seem little point, try to take pride in having clean hair, clean, ironed clothes, polished shoes and clean fingernails.

- Combat loneliness by talking to as many people as possible during the day; writing letters and making phone calls will help too.

- Consider getting a pet to bring some extra interest and companionship into your life – but only if you know you have the commitment to look after it properly.

- Take regular exercise as this triggers the secretion of natural antidepressant substances in the brain and will help to lift a low mood.

- If you find yourself thinking negative thoughts, turn them instantly into positive ones (see page 202).

- Keep a diary and at the end of each day write down what you have achieved, what you have enjoyed, and what you would like to do tomorrow to bring more happiness into your life.

- Eat plenty of fruit, vegetables, wholegrain cereals, nuts and seeds.

- Get at least half your daily calories from complex, unrefined carbohydrates such as brown rice, wholegrain cereals, wholewheat pasta and brown bread.

- Limit your intake of fats, alcohol, salt and caffeine.

- Increase your intake of foods rich in the B group vitamins such as yeast extract, wholegrains, soya, oily fish and green leafy vegetables.

- St John's wort extracts can lift low mood and improve alertness and concentration, providing relief from feelings of anxiety, agitation, disinterest, insomnia, headache and despair.

Eczema

Eczema is an inflammatory skin disease that commonly appears on the hands, inside the elbows or behind the knees but may be found anywhere on the body. Around one in ten people are affected, and most find that symptoms flare up whenever they are under stress although the cause of worry may not always be obvious, especially in children. Eczema tends to run in families and can also be triggered by allergies, exposure to certain chemicals and overgrowth of certain skin bacteria.

Eczema seems to be due to overactivity of immune cells in the skin. Scientists have recently discovered that when you are under stress, a chemical released from nerve endings in the skin affects the activity of immune cells and makes eczema symptoms worse. So, while it isn't exactly caused by stress, pressure can bring symptoms on or make them worse. Eczema symptoms can also be a cause of stress themselves. Itching, for example, is often severe enough to keep sufferers awake at night, leading to exhaustion and worsening feelings of stress. Lesions on the skin can also cause emotional distress with anxiety, feelings of embarrassment and shame, lack of confidence and low mood.

Self-help

- Take evening primrose oil supplements (1000–3000 mg) daily.

- Eat foods rich in essential fatty acids such as nuts, seeds and oily fish.

- Dilute 12 drops aromatherapy essential oils (selected from fennel, camomile, geranium, hyssop, juniper or lavender) to 50 ml carrier oil and apply to affected area twice a day (avoid during pregnancy).

- Relieve eczema symptoms with marigold tea. Make an infusion by adding 30 g marigold flowers or petals to 600 ml boiling water. Drain after 5–10 minutes and drink throughout the day. May also be used to bathe skin lesions.

- Take a good vitamin and mineral supplement containing around 100 per cent of the recommended daily amount of the following nutrients, lack of which have been linked with scaly skin problems: vitamins A, B2, B3, C, E, biotin, iodine, manganese, selenium and zinc.

- Use an emollient cream (for example, aqueous cream, dry skin cream containing evening primrose oil) to moisturize skin.

- Use aqueous cream instead of soap: substitute by simply applying to the skin, massaging in lightly then rinsing off.

- For flaky scalp, wash hair regularly with a shampoo containing tea tree oil.

- Consult a homeopath for a remedy that matches your symptoms (see page 180).

- Dead Sea salts contain minerals such as magnesium chloride, potassium chloride, sodium chloride, calcium chloride, bromides and sulphates that can help a number of scaly skin problems such as eczema. Add to bath water and soak for at least 20 minutes to help you relax. Dead Sea mud packs can also be applied to skin for a more intensive treatment.

Hair-pulling

Most people will have used the phrase, 'I'm tearing my hair out' when they are feeling under excess pressure. Few are aware that some people actually do this. Trichotillomania is closely linked with stress and is thought to affect as many as one in 50 people, making it as least as common as other, better known anxiety-related conditions such as panic attacks. Because sufferers are usually unwilling to talk about their condition through feelings of shame, hopelessness and embarrassment, few people seek help and few doctors are experienced in helping people with the condition.

People with trichotillomania may pluck hair from their scalp, eyebrows, eyelashes, legs or pubic area – anywhere, in fact, that hair is present. This leads to noticeable areas of hair loss and occasionally causes complete baldness. Most people with trichotillomania pull hair from more than one site on the body. Some may also bite their nails or pick at their skin, which may lead to scarring, disfigurement and chronic skin conditions. The hair is frequently eaten as well and can lead to a build up of a hairball (trichobezoar) in the stomach.

Often, this hair-pulling is absent-minded, done when the person is concentrating on something else such as reading or watching TV. At other times, however, the hair is pulled out with concentration and deliberation – usually when alone. The length of an attack can vary from only a few minutes to several hours. During an extreme attack, a sufferer may clear her whole head of hair within five hours.

Symptoms frequently start around the time of puberty but can occur at any age. It is rare for someone to start pulling for the first time over the age of 60, however. In childhood, boys and girls seem to be equally affected. Trichotillomania starting at puberty is from five to ten times more common in females than males and in adults seeking help there are approximately 12 females for every male. Some people with trichotillomania have other symptoms of obsessive-compulsive disorder such as compulsive checking, hand-washing or cleanliness.

Self-help

- Habit reversal training involves learning a structured method to increase awareness of the hair-pulling activity and what might trigger it, and to replace pulling with a more acceptable behavioural response so that the urge to pull is controlled. Individual, tailored treatment with a behavioural therapist is usually important for success. Group therapy may also help.

- Self-confidence can be enhanced by substituting positive, calming thoughts for those that are stressful and negative.

- Regularly say the most appropriate positive statements for you as affirmations to counter negative self-talk and feelings. If you say them frequently enough they will automatically come to mind in an emotional emergency and have a profoundly calming effect.

Headaches and migraine

Headaches are one of the most common symptoms of stress since blood-flow to the brain is affected by tension in the neck and scalp muscles, as well as by high levels of stress-related chemicals such as adrenaline.

Many people are unsure whether their stress-related symptoms are tension headaches or migraine. A tension headache tends to feel like a severe, continuous pressure on both sides of the head, which may seem to centre over the top of the skull, over the back of the head or above both eyes. Some tension headaches feel like a tight, constricting band, while others are more like a non-specific ache. In contrast, migraine pain is severe and so much worse than a tension headache that it is usually described as a full-blown attack. The pain is usually only felt on one side of the head or is definitely worse on one side.

Both migraine and tension headaches can be brought on by stress-related factors such as feelings of excess pressure, relief of stress (for example, at the end of a long, trying week), physical fatigue, lack of sleep, missed meals and extreme emotions such as anger and excitement. Migraine can also be triggered by certain foods – especially cheese, red wine and chocolate – and by hormonal changes, for example those that occur around the time of menstruation or that are associated with the oral contraceptive pill.

Self-help

- Try to work out what factors trigger your attacks and, where possible, avoid them.

- Look out for signs of tension in the way you sit and stand. Try not to stoop when standing or sitting, and concentrate on keeping your back straight, your shoulders square and your abdomen lightly pulled in. This will help to reduce feelings of stress by helping you breathe correctly using your diaphragm and abdominal muscles.

- Avoid folding your arms tightly – let your upper arms hang loosely from your shoulders, and widen the angle at your elbows.

- Hold your shoulders straight yet relaxed, and circle them from time to time to relieve any built-up tension.

- Avoid clenching your fists. Hold your hands loose with your palms open and your fingers curled lightly and naturally.

- Avoid clenching or grinding your teeth. Keep your mouth slightly open and try to relax your upper and lower jaws – every now and then open your mouth wide and move your jaw from side to side.

- Gentle manipulation of muscles in the neck, shoulders and back can help to relax taut muscles and relieve tension headaches.

- Simulation of acupoints on the stomach and large and small meridians plus use of moxibustion is often effective.

- Essential oils that can help a tension headache (do not use during pregnancy) include: camomile, geranium, lavender and peppermint.

High blood pressure

High blood pressure is common and affects as many as one in five adults. The incidence increases with age, so it becomes more common in middle life and beyond, although it can develop earlier. High blood pressure is now thought to be linked with excessive levels of stress in some people. When you are under excess stress, your blood pressure goes up by an amount equivalent to carrying an extra 40 lbs in weight, or an additional 20 years in age. Stress is intended only to produce a transient rise in blood pressure when adrenaline causes arteries and veins to constrict. In some individuals, however, the nervous system is overactive and is unusually responsive to levels of stress that would normally be associated with only a mild, temporary rise in blood pressure. This is probably an inherited trait. In people who are sensitive to the effects of stress, their blood pressure may show a tendency towards becoming high by varying considerably from time to time so it is sometimes high, sometimes low and other times normal. This is known as Gaisbock's syndrome and is a sign that if your lifestyle and levels of stress don't slow down, you may develop permanent high blood pressure (hypertension) in the future.

If your blood pressure temporarily goes very high during a stressful situation, you will not usually notice any symptoms, although a few people develop a pounding sensation in their ears or a tension headache. If your blood pressure stays high all the time and remains untreated, however, it will damage your circulation and contribute to hardening and furring up of the arteries. This in turn increases your blood pressure even more so your risk of a heart attack or stroke increases. Persistent hypertension also damages small arteries in the circulation and can lead to changes in the eyes and kidneys. Even if your blood pressure is dangerously high, you may feel relatively well. Because of this, it's worth having your blood pressure checked on a regular basis. Early diagnosis and successful treatment of high blood pressure will help to keep you healthy.

Self-help

- Lose any excess weight – shedding as little as 3–4 kg in weight can be enough to bring a moderately raised blood pressure down to normal levels again.

- If you smoke, make a concerted effort to stop – chemicals in cigarettes damage artery linings, cause spasm and constriction of vessels, and raise your blood pressure.

- Reduce your overall consumption of fat so that it makes up no more than 30 per cent of your daily energy intake – with saturated fat ideally making up no more than 15 per cent of daily calories. Eat more of the healthy fats such as olive, walnut, rapeseed and fish oils instead, which help to keep the circulation healthy.

- Eat plenty of fresh fruit and vegetables for protective vitamins, minerals and fibre.

- Keep alcohol intake within recommended limits.

- Increase the amount of exercise you take.

- If you are diabetic, make sure your blood sugar levels are well controlled.

- Consider taking an antioxidant supplement which may protect against hardening and furring up of the arteries. The most important dietary antioxidants are vitamins A/betacarotene, C, E and selenium.

- Essential oils that can help lower high blood pressure (do not use during pregnancy) include: clary sage, geranium, lavender, lemon, marjoram, melissa and nutmeg.

- Yoga is excellent for improving joint suppleness, relieving stress and reducing high blood pressure.

- Dandelion is a diuretic used to help flush excess salts and fluid through the kidneys. It is a useful treatment for high blood pressure as it can reduce fluid retention without also encouraging a build-up of sodium.

- Garlic-powder tablets can lower high blood pressure, high cholesterol levels and blood stickiness enough to reduce the risk of a stroke by almost a half, and the risk of a coronary heart disease by a quarter.

Impotence

Impotence – also known as erectile dysfunction – affects as many as one in ten men on a regular basis. It is especially common in men who are under stress, since anxiety interferes with the normal processes of arousal. Stress can also lead to smoking and the long-term abuse of alcohol or recreational drugs, which can also affect male potency.

As well as being a sign of stress, impotence is also a powerful cause of stress – one in five men with erectile dysfunction blame impotence for the break-up of their relationships, for example. This can set up yet another vicious stress circle, so it is important to seek help sooner rather than later.

Self-help

- More than nine out of ten men are able to regain potency with one of the many treatments now available such as psychosexual coun- selling, drug treatments (for example Viagra, testosterone replacement therapy, penile injections), mechanical aids (vacuum pumps, implants) and vascular surgery to improve circulation.

- Ginkgo biloba extracts can relax blood vessels to boost circulation to the brain, hands, feet and genitals. It can increase blood flow to the penis: half of previously impotent men have regained full potency after taking it for six months. (See also page 151.)

- Bach Flower Rescue Remedy can be helpful for men fearing impotence or poor performance.

Indigestion and heartburn

People under stress have increased activity in the nerve endings supplying the stomach. This can lead to increased secretion of acidic juices and churning sensations (butterflies) due to increased muscular contraction of the stomach. This is linked with symptoms of heartburn (acid reflux from the stomach up into the oesophagus) and peptic ulcers in the stomach or duodenum.

Indigestion and heartburn are common and unpleasant symptoms linked with eating and are especially common when you are under excessive stress. Symptoms include feelings of distension from swallowing air, flatulence from excessive wind in the intestines, nausea, abdominal pain and sensations of burning. Indigestion (or dyspepsia) is the term used to describe discomfort or burning felt centrally in the upper abdomen, while heartburn is the term used for discomfort felt behind the chest bone (sternum).

One of the most common causes of heartburn is acid reflux, in which stomach contents reflux up into the oesophagus – the tube connecting the mouth and stomach. Normally this is prevented by a muscle sphincter, and by downward contractions of muscles in the gut wall. This protective mechanism may fail due to poor muscle coordination, weakness of the stomach sphincter, the presence of a hiatus hernia, or increased pressure on the stomach, for example due to excess weight or overeating.

Self-help

- Eat little and often throughout the day, rather than having three large meals.
- Drink fluids little and often, rather than large quantities at a time.
- Avoid hot, acid, spicy, fatty foods.
- Avoid tea, coffee and acidic fruit juices.
- Cut back on alcohol intake.
- Avoid aspirin and related drugs (for example, ibuprofen) if you are prone to indigestion – if necessary, take paracetamol instead.
- Avoid stooping, bending or lying down after eating.
- Avoid late-night eating.
- Elevate the head of the bed about 15–20 cm (for example, put books under the legs at that end).
- Wear loose clothing, especially around the waist.
- Drink milk or take an antacid to help ease burning sensations.
- Longer-term measures to help control your symptoms include losing any excess weight and not smoking cigarettes.

Infections

More than 200 different viruses can cause symptoms of the common cold. Researchers have found that high levels of stress double the chance of developing symptoms when exposed to a cold virus. This is most likely when you feel tired and 'run down' and is thought to be due to stress hormones interfering with immune function in some way.

Self-help

- To help boost your natural immunity, eat a healthy, wholefood and preferably organic diet that provides at least five servings of fruit and vegetables per day (see Chapter 4).

- Eat as much fruit, vegetables and salad-stuff raw as possible to preserve their immune-boosting plant substances (phytochemicals).

- While diet should always come first, a good multinutrient supplement provides a nutritional safety net. Choose one containing around 100 per cent of the recommended daily amount (RDA) of as many vitamins and minerals as possible. Even a relatively minor lack of some nutrients can lower your immunity.

- Try to eat oily fish (for example salmon, mackerel, herring, sardines) at least once or twice a week. These contain essential fatty acids important for good immune function. If you don't like eating fish, consider taking an omega-3 supplement. Evening primrose oil capsules supply important essential fatty acids, too.

- Take vitamin C (at least 1,000 mg daily) with bioflavonoids to help to protect against viral infections, and if symptoms of a cold start to develop, suck throat lozenges containing zinc – these boost the action of white blood cells in the throat and can reduce symptoms of the common cold.

- Take regular exercise (see Chapter 4).

- Take time out to relax (see Chapter 4).

- Get a regular good night's sleep (see page 71).

- Many herbal remedies are known to boost immunity. Results are often greatest when used together with vitamin C and a vitamin B complex. Popular immune boosters include aloe vera, astragalus, echinacea, garlic powder tablets, gotu kola and Korean, Chinese, American and Siberian ginsengs (see Chapter 3 for more information).

Insomnia

Stress is the most common cause of lack of sleep and, in turn, lack of sleep is a common cause of stress. Once you develop insomnia, stress and lack of sleep can keep feeding on each other to make each condition worse.

Sleep is a form of unconsciousness that is our natural state of rest. It is the strongest instinctive urge in humans, yet scientists still do not fully understand how or why we sleep although they do know it is essential for our continued physical and emotional well-being. We are designed to spend around a third of our life asleep, yet four out of ten people do not get a regular good night's rest. As a result, they wake up feeling tired, make more mistakes during the day, and may repeatedly fall asleep for several seconds at a time. These so-called microsleeps are a common cause of accidents, both on the roads and in the home.

Most people have suffered from insomnia at some stage of their life – usually when they are worried or stressed. Stress can cause difficulty in falling asleep, tossing and turning without finding a comfortable position, difficulty staying asleep, and waking up feeling unrefreshed. Recurrent lack of sleep leads to poor performance and achievement during the day. Insomnia is also linked with increased risk of serious stress-related illness such as high blood pressure, stroke and even a heart attack.

Stress-related insomnia may be: transient (lasting only a few days), short-term (lasting 1–3 months) or long-term (lasting over 3 months).

Caffeine, stress and sleep

Caffeine – found in tea, coffee, chocolate, soft drinks such as colas, and some over-the-counter analgesic blends – is a stimulant drug whose immediate effect is to reduce tiredness and make the body feel alert. Coffee is often consumed in large amounts (eight to ten cups a day, for example) when you are under pressure, and this can make symptoms of stress even worse. As it is also a stimulant, it interferes with sleeping even more.

High intakes of caffeine may cause withdrawal symptoms such as irritability, cravings and increased stress when you try to reduce them. If you think you are drinking too much coffee, reduce your intake by switching to decaffeinated brands. If stopping caffeine suddenly seems to be making you jittery, gradually reduce your intake by replacing every other cup with a decaffeinated brand, slowly reducing your intake further.

Self-help

- Avoid napping during the day as this will make it more difficult to sleep at night.
- Take regular exercise, as active peope tend to sleep more easily.
- Eat a healthy, low-fat, wholefood diet with plenty of complex carbo-hydrates and fruit and vegetables (see Chapter 3).

- Try to eat your evening meal before 7pm and resist late-night snacks, especially of rich food.

- A warm, milky drink just before going to bed will help you to relax – hot milk with cinnamon or nutmeg is better than chocolate drinks, which contain some caffeine. Don't drink too much fluid in the evening, however – a full bladder is guaranteed to disturb your rest.

- If you can't sleep, don't lie there tossing and turning. Get up and read or watch the television for a while. If you are worried about something, write down all the things on your mind and promise yourself you will deal with them in the morning, when you are feeling fresher. When you feel sleepy, go back to bed and try again.

- Try alternative therapies such as acupuncture, reflexology and meditation (see Chapter 5).

- Herbal supplements containing natural extracts of three herbs: valerian (*Valeriana officinalis*), lemon balm (*Melissa officinalis*) and hops (*Humulus lupulus*) can induce a refreshing night's sleep without the side effects associated with drugs (see also Chapter 3).

- Soothing herbal teas can also help you sleep. Try infusions of lime-flower, lemon balm, fennel, rosehips, passionflower, nutmeg, cinnamon, camomile, valerian or skullcap. It is also worth investing in a herbal pillow filled with dried lavender flowers to place at the head of your bed.

- Consult a homeopath for a remedy that matches your symptoms (see page 180).

- Try some Bach Flower Remedies (see page 177).

- Aromatherapy can improve sleep problems dramatically (only use under specialist advice during pregnancy). Add five drops of essential oil to 10 ml (2 teaspoons) almond oil and pour into a deep, warm – not hot – bath. Relax in the fragrant water for 15–20 minutes, then sprinkle a few drops of the same essential oil on a cottonwool pad and tuck under your pillow. Choose your favourite fragrance from: camomile, geranium, juniper, lavender, neroli, rose, sandalwood and ylang-ylang. Mix several oils together in blends if you prefer. Vary the oils every four to five days, otherwise you will adapt to them and treatment will be less effective.

- Chiropractors manipulate the spine with rapid, direct thrusts to correct poor alignment. If sleep is difficult because of tension in your neck, or shoulder or back pain, a chiropractor can manipulate your back to realign muscles, tendons, ligaments, joints and bones to ease tension and help you to relax.

- A hypnotherapist will help to uncover subconscious fears and anxieties that are causing stress, then uses suggestions to help you relax, lose your fears and sleep more easily. Suggestions can be taped and replayed when you go to bed.

- There are many different types of massage that use a variety of rubbing, drumming, kneading, friction and pressure strokes. All are very relaxing. Therapeutic massage is particularly useful in helping sleep problems due to stress and muscle tension, especially when combined with aromatherapy essential oils.

Irritability

Everyone becomes irritable from time to time when they are tired, especially if they haven't eaten properly or skipped a meal and their blood-sugar level is low. Irritability can also be a feature of premenstrual syndrome (see page 121), menopausal symptoms (see page 117) and other forms of internal or external stress. When you realize you are being irritable, try to take steps to improve your mood before it gets any worse.

Self-help

- Say 'Calm!' quietly to yourself and practise a breathing exercise.

- Keep a pack of dried fruit or rice cakes at hand and have a healthy snack if irritability is likely to be linked with low blood sugar levels.

- Take a brief break from what you are doing, even if it is just to visit the bathroom – exercise will help to boost your circulation so your brain receives more oxygen, energy and vital nutrients.

- Visualize the person or situation that makes you irritable passing right through you and leaving you unaffected.

- Try to identify people or situations that regularly tend to irritate you and work out why.

- Eat regular meals – never skip breakfast or lunch.

- Avoid excess caffeine or nicotine.

- When all else fails, count silently to ten.

Alcohol and stress

When feeling stressed, it is common to feel 'I must have a drink' and for your alcohol intake to increase. Up to a certain point, alcohol seems to be beneficial, in that a moderate intake – especially of red wine – has been shown to lower a high blood pressure, reduce stress levels and decrease your risk of coronary heart disease by as much as 25–45 per cent. This is mostly due to the powerful antioxidants found in red wine, and the thinning effect of alcohol on the blood. In fact, new research suggests that if you have high blood pressure and drink within the recommended limits, your risk of dying from a stroke is 40 per cent less than for a teetotaller. These benefits of moderate intakes of alcohol are thought to be linked with the fact that those who drink are more likely to laugh and giggle than non-drinkers. Laughter helps to buffer the effects of stress and can also improve immunity and increase resistance to disease.

There is a cut-off point at which the benefits of alcohol intake are lost and excess alcohol intake is harmful to health, however. Once this point is reached, your risk of high blood pressure, coronary heart disease and stroke reverses and becomes significantly increased. At the same time, the risk of liver damage leading to cirrhosis also rises. It is therefore important not to let your alcohol intake rise above that which may be beneficial for health, no matter how stressed you feel, as this will magnify the harmful effects of the stress itself.

Healthy drinking guidelines therefore suggest that:

- Men should aim to drink no more than 3–4 units of alcohol per day. Consistently drinking 4 or more units a day is not advised, however.

- Women should drink no more than 2–3 units per day and consistently drinking 3 or more units a day is not advised. Women who are pregnant or planning a baby should aim to avoid alcohol altogether.

You should also aim to have one or two alcohol-free days per week. For men, drinking more than 50 units of alcohol per week is considered dangerous, while for women, the equivalent figure is 35 units. Most people tend to overestimate the strength of spirits and underestimate the strength of beer. It is important to realize that:

- Someone drinking two pints of beer has consumed four units.

- Someone drinking two glasses of wine and a double vodka has also consumed four units.

Simple tips to help you cut your alcohol intake:

- When drinking alcohol, sip slowly and keep putting your glass down rather than holding it in your hand – this will reduce the amount you sip out of habit, when talking.

- Savour each sip and hold it in your mouth for longer.

- Alternate each alcoholic drink with a non-alcoholic one.

- Many bars offer exotic, non-alcoholic cocktails that are delicious and full of nutrients.

- Drink mineral water with a dash of fresh lemon juice, or low-calorie drinks.

- Tonic water with ice, lemon and a dash of Angostura bitters is an excellent substitute for a gin and tonic.

- Mix chilled white or red wine with sparkling mineral water to make a refreshing spritzer.

- Elderflower cordial diluted with mineral water is an excellent substitute for white wine.

- Drink fruit/herbal teas – these are delicious, relaxing or stimulating depending on which you choose and, as they are drunk without milk, have the additional bonus of being calorie-free.

- Practise saying, 'No thanks, I'm cutting back for my health/blood pressure' or 'No thanks, alcohol and stress don't mix well together,' or, 'No thanks, I'm driving.' There is no shame in wanting to cut back the amount of alcohol you drink and your firm stand may well help someone else decide to do the same.

Irritable bowel syndrome

Irritable bowel syndrome (IBS) and stress are closely linked. Stress is not a recognized cause of IBS but it does make symptoms worse, and can bring on an attack in those who already suffer from the condition. IBS may therefore be a sign of excess stress in those who are affected.

During the body's fight-or-flight stress response, several powerful chemicals are released that affect the bowel and trigger bowel contraction. These effects stem from the need to rapidly empty the bowel to make you lighter for action. In people without IBS, these normal responses do not seem to trigger any unpleasant symptoms except for the expected diarrhoea. In those with IBS, however, the response seems to be accentuated and prolonged.

IBS is the most common condition to affect the gut and affects at least a third of the population at some time during their life, even if only mildly. IBS is a problem of bowel function rather than structure, and as a result there is nothing abnormal to find during investigations and no obvious clues to help with the diagnosis. Many sufferers find that their symptoms improve with time and disappear in later life.

Self-help

- Don't rush meals – leave plenty of time to eat so you don't bolt down your food and swallow too much air.
- Take regular exercise – this stimulates production of the body's own natural painkillers as well as relieving bloating and distension.

- Make a point of sitting down to eat rather than eating on the move.
- Try to eat little and often during the day rather than the traditional three large meals.
- Eat more complex, unrefined carbohydrates that contain a variety of fibre types such as wholegrain bread, wholemeal pasta, brown rice and unsweetened wholegrain breakfast cereals such as muesli or porridge. Cut out all pre-packaged or processed foods.
- Eat more fresh fruit and vegetables – especially nuts, seeds, figs, apricots, prunes, peas, sweetcorn and beans.
- Eat live bio yoghurt (containing a culture of *Lactobacillus acidophilus*), drink liquid yogurt containing *Lactobacillus casei* 'Shirota' (Yakult) or take acidophilus supplements to line your bowel with friendly bacteria.
- Bran fibre helps some people with IBS but not others – regularly alternate different fibre supplements such as bran, ispaghula, psyllium or sterculia as bowel bacteria quickly adapt to them and the beneficial effects may be lost.
- Eat more fish and skinless white meat rather than red meat.
- If wind is a problem, avoid beans, cabbage and any other foods that encourage bacterial fermentation and may trigger intestinal gas.
- Many natural herbs and spices contain substances that calm the bowels, relieve spasm and prevent a build up of wind. These include aniseed, camomile, lemon balm, dill, fennel, black pepper,

marjoram, parsley, peppermint, rosemary and spearmint. Use them as a garnish on food or as soothing, herbal teas.

- Drink more fluids – especially bottled water or herbal teas. Aim to drink 2–3 litres of fluid throughout the day.

- Acupuncture stimulates the release of natural painkillers, which can help to reduce the symptoms of irritable bowel syndrome, including constipation, diarrhoea and cramping pains.

- Abdominal massage can help constipation, wind and distension, as well as relieving pain associated with diarrhoea. Dilute a total of 10–20 drops of rosemary and/or marjoram essential oils in a carrier such as almond oil. Gently massage into your abdomen using firm, circular movements of one hand. NB substitute rose oil for rosemary oil if you have high blood pressure; do not use during pregnancy.

- Take ginger to reduce flatulence, nausea and colic. Peppermint or camomile tea can relieve mild intestinal cramps or flatulence. Garlic-powder tablets are helpful for diarrhoea, wind and indigestion. Aloe vera juice can relieve indigestion and constipation. Goldenseal helps to normalize bowel function, so is helpful for both constipation and diarrhoea. Ginseng is an adaptogen that can help you adapt to stress so symptoms become less troublesome.

- Hypnotherapy can significantly reduce abdominal pain and distension, encourage a regular bowel and improve general well-being.

Memory

Your memory is a personal storehouse of information. When you are under stress, however, it is natural for your memory to become less like a filing cabinet and more like a sieve. Anxiety interferes with memory storage and recall: your concentration goes and you're distracted by worry and preoccupied with personal thoughts.

Self-help

- When you want to remember an important fact, keep repeating it silently to yourself.

- Write memory-jogging notes of things to do on post-it pads and stick them up where you will easily see them.

- Associate a fact to be remembered with a visual image, for example, when introduced to someone who is an artist, picture them holding an enormous paint brush. If their name is Baker, picture them eating a large loaf of bread. The more outrageous or unusual your images, the easier you will remember them.

- If you can't remember someone's name, try to remember where you met them, what they were wearing, any unusual physical character-istic or mannerism – this will often jog your memory.

- Try to think up a mnemonic involving the first letter of each word when remembering a list. A good example is the mnemonic used to remember the colours of a rainbow: Richard of York gave battle in vain (red, orange, yellow, green, blue, indigo, violet). It is easier to remember the sentence and work out the colours, than to remember the colours alone.

- If you keep losing something, try to form a mental photograph of where they are every time you put them down.

- When trying to remember a number, use visual images (for example, a shoe for two, a gate for eight, a bottle of wine for nine).

- Eat a healthy, wholefood diet with plenty of fresh fruit, vegetables, cereals and fish – avoid processed foods containing additives as much as possible.

- Increase your intake of foods rich in vitamin B1, such as brewer's yeast, brown rice, wheatgerm, wholegrain bread and cereals.

- Eat more fish: it contains phosphatidylcholine that helps memory.

- Eat more garlic and consider taking garlic tablets to improve blood-flow through small blood vessels in the brain.

- Consider taking extracts from the *Ginkgo biloba* tree, which improve blood-flow to the brain and can improve memory and concentration.

- If you smoke, try to stop.

- Cut right back on alcohol intake.

- Increase the amount of exercise you take to boost circulation to the brain.

- Make sure you get plenty of rest and sleep.

Phobias

A phobia is a disorder associated with anxiety in which a morbid fear of certain objects or situations develops that is out of all proportion to the threat the object or situation really presents. Typically, someone with a phobia will go to any length to avoid exposure to the object or situation feared. It is estimated that as many as one in four women and one in six men have a simple phobia which, although mild, may be sufficient to interfere with some aspects of their work or lifestyle.

When you are under extreme stress, even a simple phobia can escalate until you develop a panic attack. This is such a frightening experience that you may then develop a fear of having another if you are exposed to the same situation again in the future. Eventually, this fear may broaden until you reach a stage where you cannot face meeting new people, visiting any crowded place or even going out alone. In many cases, these fears are not so much the fear of open, crowded spaces or of people themselves, but the fear of having nothing interesting to say, not being able to cope or of looking foolish by having a panic attack in public.

Self-help

- A simple phobia can be treated with behaviour therapy in which gradual desensitization slowly exposes the sufferer to the object feared. The first exposure to the feared situation is obviously very stressful and will make you feel very anxious and stressed. If you stay in the situation and try to view it rationally, however, your anxiety will slowly decrease. Each time you confront the fear again, you will usually find your level of anxiety decreases and you recover your composure more quickly.

- Try to realize that the situation or object you fear is relatively harmless. Write down all the worst things you fear might happen to you if you faced your fear. Go back over each of these and plan how you could cope with each of these situations in a cool, calm and collected manner.

- Close your eyes, relax, then slowly visualize yourself in the situation you fear. Try to stay with the image for longer and longer each day, then imagine yourself confronting the fear, calmly walking past it and leaving it totally behind.

- Obtain a picture of the situation or object that you fear and practise looking at it and handling it for longer and longer periods each day.

- Discuss your feelings and fears openly with other people and listen to theirs – this form of group therapy can be very helpful.

- Arrange to expose yourself to the fear with someone you trust – a best friend, partner or close relative. It is often easier to face your fears initially while holding someone else's hand for moral support.

- Develop positive statements of self-worth (see page 202).

- Hypnotherapy (see page 184) is especially effective for treating phobias. In a typical group session you will be helped to achieve a relaxed state and shown how to use visualization and auto-suggestion to help overcome your irrational fear.

Psoriasis

Psoriasis is a skin condition in which skin cells are produced ten times faster than normal. New skin cells push to the surface in around seven days rather than the more usual 28, which causes a build-up of cells to produce silver-white thickened plaques with an underlying redness due to dilated blood vessels.

Psoriasis affects around one in 50 adults. It tends to run in families with skin lesions commonly appearing on the knees, elbows and scalp. Between 10 and 20 per cent of people with psoriasis also develop a form of arthritis known as psoriatic arthropathy.

The exact cause of psoriasis is unknown, but flare-ups are closely related to stress. Many sufferers find their symptoms flare up when they are under stress, for example taking examinations, following bereavement, serious marital or financial problems or the shock of illness/accidents. It is also common for psoriasis to occur for the first time after a stressful situation, including infections, trauma and childbirth. Symptoms can also be made worse by smoking, drinking excess alcohol and, in some cases, by exposure to sunlight and cold weather.

Self-help

- Avoid stress as much as possible.
- Take evening primrose oil supplements (1000–3000 mg) daily.
- Eat foods rich in essential fatty acids such as nuts, seeds and oily fish.

- When applying topical therapy to the body, sit with the skin uncovered for at least 15 minutes, then put on loose clothing so the preparation is not rubbed off. When waiting for medication applied to the skin to soak in, practise breathing exercises and other relaxation techniques (see page 154).

- If the area needs washing (for example, hands, elbows, feet), give a topical agent enough time to penetrate (at least 15 minutes) and use this time to practise positive self-affirmations (see page 202).

- When applying treatment to the scalp, apply thoroughly at least an hour before going to bed so the medication doesn't rub off on to the pillow before having time to work; wearing a disposable shower cap for at least an hour helps treatment penetration. While waiting for treatment to soak in, practise a visualization technique (see page 193) in which you imagine your skin lesions melting away.

- Use an emollient cream (for example, aqueous cream, emulsifying ointment, dry skin cream containing evening primrose oil) to moisturize your skin.

- Use aqueous cream instead of soap: substitute by simply applying to the skin, massaging in lightly, then rinsing off.

- Use a bath emollient to soothe, hydrate and soften the skin.

- Aloe vera gel or cream can improve psoriasis lesions by over 80 per cent.

- Fish oil supplements in liquid or capsule form seem to help in 15–50 per cent of people with psoriasis.

Restless legs syndrome

Restless legs syndrome causes an unpleasant creeping sensation in the lower limbs accompanied by twitching, pins and needles, burning sensations and a sudden, irresistible urge to move your legs. This relieves symptoms only fleetingly before the irresistible urge returns. The desire to move your legs may keep waking you when you are tired and trying to drift off to sleep. Restless legs syndrome affects around one in 20 people regularly and tends to occur when you are suffering from fatigue, anxiety or stress.

Self-help

- Take a vitamin and mineral supplement that includes iron, folic acid and vitamin E.
- Consider taking coenzyme Q10 – a vitamin-like substance that increases oxygen uptake in cells.
- Just before going to sleep, try placing your feet in cold water for five minutes to help promote sleep.
- Avoid synthetic socks, tights and underwear as these seem to make the condition worse.
- Avoid alcohol and caffeine, which may make symptoms worse.
- A gel developed for tired legs, which contains extracts of seaweed, hazel, grape, butcher's-broom, pine, camphor and lavender, is said to improve symptoms in more than three-quarters of patients.

Sex drive

Sexual problems are common among people experiencing excess pressure. Loss of sex drive is especially likely and affects at least 60 per cent of adults under stress, 30 per cent of middle-aged women and over 70 per cent of post-menopausal women. Stress-related loss of sex drive is largely due to hormone changes produced as a result of a prolonged fight-or-flight response.

Stress is one of the most widespread causes of loss of sex drive, or libido, along with overwork, tiredness and lack of sleep. Excess stress is associated with a fall in testosterone and oestrogen levels, and an increase in secretion of prolactin – a hormone produced by the pituitary gland in the brain. Prolactin has a powerful negative effect on libido, and literally switches off the sex drive as well as reducing fertility. Low sex drive is in itself a powerful cause of stress in relationships, so a vicious circle sets up. It is therefore important to tackle low sex drive sooner rather than later.

Self-help

- Start taking steps to lose any excess weight by eating more healthily.
- Exercise regularly to build up your stamina.
- Reduce your intake of alcohol to within safe limits.
- Improve your self-esteem (see Chapter 6).
- Make sure you get a regular good night's sleep.

- Take a vitamin and mineral supplement to help correct any deficiencies.

- Korean and American Ginsengs can help the body adapt to physical and emotional stress and are widely reputed to have an aphrodisiac effect. Siberian ginseng is also noted for its aphrodisiac properties.

- St John's wort helps 60 per cent of post-menopausal women become interested in sex again after three months of treatment.

- Consult a homeopath for a remedy that matches your symptoms (see page 180).

- The heavy, floral essential oils of geranium, rose, jasmine and ylang-ylang are among the most powerful aromatic aphrodisiacs. Other essential oils that can increase sex drive include black pepper, cardamom, cinnamon (for perfuming the air only – do not bring into contact with the skin) and ginger.

Smoking and stress

During times of stress, it is common for smokers to increase the number of cigarettes they smoke. This is a subconscious behavioural response since nicotine produces a drug-like soothing effect on the nervous system. However, nicotine also acts on the body to produce symptoms similar to some of those occurring in the stress fight-or-flight response such as muscle tension, tremor and jitteriness, as well as affecting bowel function. Smoking is also linked with sex hormone imbalances – smokers' fertility falls and women who smoke are likely to enter the menopause up to two years earlier than non-smokers – not to mention the fact that smoking is a powerful cause of premature skin ageing and wrinkles.

Cigarette smoke contains over 4000 different chemicals, many of which are harmful and cancer forming. These chemicals damage the lining of arteries to increase the risk of them hardening and furring up, high blood pressure, coronary heart disease and stroke as well as affecting cell division to increase the risk of cancer. Smoking therefore maximizes many of the harmful effects produced by prolonged, excessive stress. If you are stressed and smoke, one of the greatest contributions you can make to your long-term health is to stop smoking.

If you can give up:

● Within 20 minutes your blood pressure and pulse rate will fall significantly as arterial spasm decreases.

1

- Within 48 hours the stickiness of your blood and the quantity of blood clotting factors present will fall enough to reduce your risk of a heart attack or stroke.

- Within one to three months the blood supply to your peripheries will increase, and your lung function will improve by up to a third.

- Within five years your risk of lung cancer will have halved.

- Within ten years your risk of all smoking-related cancers (for example, lung, mouth, throat, bladder) will have reduced to almost normal levels.

Giving up is not easy when you are also having to cope with excess pressure, however. Nicotine is addictive, which is why it is so difficult to quit. Withdrawal symptoms of tension, aggression, depression, insomnia and cravings can occur, which will magnify the psychological and emotional effects of any stress you are under. A 'quit plan' to help you stop smoking is outlined here. Your doctor will be pleased to help you, too.

Tips to help you stop smoking:

- Find support – giving up nicotine is easier with a friend or partner.

- Name the day to cut back or give up and get into the right frame of mind. If cutting back, cut out a number of cigarettes per day, starting with those you will miss the least. Then continue reducing your intake until you gradually stop, or until you feel ready to cut out the remaining cigarettes altogether.

- Get rid of temptation. Throw away all smoking papers, matches, lighters, ashtrays, spare packets, etc. before the day arrives.

- When you want to smoke, instead of saying, 'I must have a cigarette,' change your thought patterns and say instead, 'While I would like a cigarette, I don't need one because I no longer smoke,' then remind yourself of all the reasons you have decided to quit.

- Keep a quit chart and tick off every day you keep within your target level of consumption or have lasted without a cigarette. Plan a reward for every week of success.

- Learn to relax. Have a massage, practise yoga or meditation. You need something to replace the anxiety-relieving effects of nicotine.

- Find a hobby to take your mind off smoking – a habit that keeps your hands busy is best – and keep active with DIY jobs in the evening rather than sitting in front of the TV.

- Increase the amount of regular exercise you take as this can help to curb withdrawal symptoms.

- Identify situations where you would usually smoke and either avoid them or plan ahead to overcome them, for example practise saying, 'No thanks, I've given up,' or 'No thanks, I'm cutting down.'

- Ask friends and relatives not to smoke around you.

- Watch your diet. Avoid excess saturated fats and count calories so you don't put on weight. Chew sugar-free gum or drink water and unsweetened herbal teas instead.

- Save the money previously spent on cigarettes to buy a luxury for yourself or to spend on a happiness retreat or a stress-busting weekend break.

Tired all the time (TATT)

Occasional tiredness is normal, and affects everyone, but increasing numbers of people admit to feeling tired all the time – usually shortened to TATT. This is one of the most common physical symptoms to accompany prolonged excess pressure and tends to creep up on you, making you feel washed out and exhausted for much of the time. Interestingly, more women than men are affected, perhaps because women are much more likely to juggle different aspects of their life – looking after the home, working, raising children, organizing meals – and have less time to sit down, put their feet up and look after their own health. Surveys suggest that as many as three out of four women feel constantly tired, with the majority naming stress as the major cause.

When TATT is persistent and affects the quality of your life, it is important to learn to control it. TATT can often be overcome by improving your diet, improving the quality of your sleep and increasing the amount of exercise you take.

Self-help

- You'll be surprised how much better you will feel if you eat a healthy, low-fat diet full of wholegrain cereals, fresh fruit and vegetables.

- Lack of vitamins and minerals can make TATT worse. The B-group of vitamins are especially important.

- Make sure you obtain enough iron in your diet. One in three women are anaemic due to menstruation, pregnancy, poor diet or poor ability to absorb and store iron (see page 71).

- Avoid excess caffeine (see page 71).

- Lack of sleep increases feelings of TATT as sleep is a time of rest, repair, rejuvenation and regeneration. It allows your body to rest and your muscles and joints to recover from constant use during the day. Cell turnover rate increases and more red blood cells and immune cells are made (see page 71 for tips on getting a better night's rest).

- Exercise regularly, as it is important to get fit. Apart from encouraging your body to become overweight, lack of exercise can cause lack of energy and feeling tired all the time – and can also lower your mood.

- Find time for relaxation. Treat yourself to a massage, a facial, or a soak in an aromatherapy bath. Just sitting quietly and listening to music or finding a quiet spot to read a book will help. Encourage the family not to disturb you during your relaxation period.

If you feel tired all the time for longer than two weeks, despite increasing your exercise levels, eating a healthy diet and improving your quality of sleep, consult your doctor. Many illnesses start off with tiredness as one of their first symptoms. While most people who feel tired are unlikely to be seriously ill, it's still worth having a check-up just in case. This is especially important if you have also noticed other symptoms such as weight loss, cough, shortness of breath, urinary problems or thirst.

TMJ Syndrome

Stress is a common cause of TMJ syndrome, which affects the temporomandibular joint (TMJ) between the jawbone and skull. The joint is unusual in that it contains a disc of cartilage that provides a smooth internal articular surface and increases the range of movement of the jaw.

TMJ syndrome is often linked with excess tension and spasm in the chewing muscles in people who are stressed, or who subconsciously clench their teeth when feeling under excess pressure. TMJ syndrome can also be caused by the habit of holding a telephone receiver between your shoulder and cheek, and by an incorrect tooth alignment.

TMJ syndrome is associated with a range of symptoms that may not all occur in everyone: headache, tender jaw muscles, aching pain around the face, difficulty in opening the mouth, locking of the jaw and clicking as the jaw is opened or closed (this is quite common and when it occurs alone does not necessarily mean you have TMJ syndrome).

Self-help

- Consult a dentist, who will check your bite, your muscles and your jaw's range of movement.
- Rest the joint, apply warmth and follow a soft diet to help reduce spasm of chewing muscles.
- Devices to prevent clenching or grinding the teeth at night are available – ask your dentist for advice.

2 DISCOVER THE CAUSES OF STRESS

As already discussed, some pressure in life is normal and necessary, and only becomes harmful when it is excessive or prolonged, at which stage the feelings you experience are known as stress. One of the most important steps in managing the pressures in your life is to recognize the ones that are potential sources of stress for you. These are known as your stressors. Having recognized your stressors, you then need to weigh them up to see how severe a threat they really are compared with how bad you believe them to be. Your perceptions of threat play a key role in the way you react and it is a common tendency to overestimate problems. Feelings of stress feed on each other and can produce unpleasant sensations of panic. These can, in turn, lead to fears or phobias that may seem irrational on the surface but feel very real deep down. It is often the people who appear most cool under pressure who are most vulnerable to anxiety and stress – this is because they fear losing control, which magnifies many of the challenges they meet.

Internal and external causes

Sources of stress rarely exist in isolation and it is common for several related events to combine to produce feelings of excess pressure. It is important to try to identify what these are so you can plan how to start removing them from your life. The sources of your stress can be either internal, within you, or external, caused by events outside you.

The speed of these changes will play an important part in determining whether or not you feel stressed. Slow changes give you a chance to gradually adjust and become familiar with new experiences. In this way you can acquire new coping skills without being aware of undue pressure. Rapid changes are the most stressful, since the goal posts seem to be moving in front of your eyes and it is difficult to fully assess what is happening, let alone prepare in advance for the impact these changes may have on your life.

Although external factors may be the stimulus for the stress you are experiencing (see box, page 99), it is usually how you react to these changes that actually results in your feelings of stress. Type B personalities will react very differently from Type As, for example, so although you may feel your stress is totally due to pressures from outside you, most sensations of stress are in fact self-generated.

Internal causes of stress

There are many internal causes of stress. These include certain personality traits, such as the competitive Type A discussed previously, uncertainty about your goals in life and having a negative self-image. Have a look at the following internal causes of stress and tick all those that are relevant to you:

- The physical and emotional effects of working long hours
- Inadequate time off for relaxation
- Lack of sleep
- Physical tiredness
- Mental exhaustion
- Menstruation
- Menopause
- Negative self-image
- Negative thoughts
- Lack of fitness
- Disruption of bio-rhythms caused by such things as shift work, jet lag and insomnia
- Physical or mental ill-health

External causes of stress

Sources of external stress are mainly related to change, since anything new readily evokes a stress response to help you prepare for the unknown challenge. Change causes uncertainty, uncertainty leads to anxiety and anxiety is a powerful trigger for stress. Different changes therefore set up a chain reaction of similar responses, whether they are related to changes in your relationships with other people, changes in family dynamics or changes occurring at work. Have a look at the following list and tick all those where changes are currently happening in your life:

- [ ] Changes in your relationship with your husband/wife/girlfriend/ boyfriend
- [ ] Changes in your job title/position
- [ ] Changes in your working environment
- [ ] Changes in your career prospects. Changes in your relationships with work colleagues
- [ ] Changes in your hours of work
- [ ] Changing from working to retirement or redundancy
- [ ] Changes in your living accommodation
- [ ] Changes in your health
- [ ] Changes in your relationships with relatives
- [ ] Changes in your social life/relationships with friends
- [ ] Changes in your hobbies/recreations

The exceptions are environmental situations, which tend to cause stress for everyone, such as excessive heat, cold, humidity or prolonged exposure to loud noise or bright lights.

The way you respond to change depends largely on whether you perceive the changes as desirable or a threat. If you see the changes as desirable, the feelings you experience will remain on the level of positive pressure. If you see the changes as a threat, however, then you are programmed to start experiencing feelings of stress. The degree of stress you feel in turn reflects how well you think you can cope.

Changes that are perceived as desirable are often those you have deliberately instigated yourself – for example, moving house, changing jobs or finishing an unrewarding relationship. If these same changes were imposed on you – having to move house because of your job, having your job description restructured or being deserted by your partner – the situation would be entirely different. Change plus the feeling that you have little control over a difficult situation causes frustration and strong negative feelings against the changes themselves and those who have instigated them. These will inevitably trigger feelings of stress.

Analysing change

It is often helpful to analyse possible changes in your life in terms of whether they are desirable or a threat, chosen or imposed, to work out in advance how stressful they are likely to be. You may think that few changes are likely to be both chosen and a threat, but in fact those who are most successful in life are often those who deliberately choose to face extremely challenging situations, such as climbing Mount Everest or volunteering for public speaking. Success and the acquisition of new life-skills often comes from daring to do what others fear or refuse to do.

You therefore need to be realistic about exactly how each change (chosen or imposed) is likely to impact on your life. Few changes or sources of stress exist in isolation and it is important to consider all the knock-on effects they will produce when assessing the degree of threat or desirable challenge they represent.

Internal causes of stress are generally easier to deal with than external problems, because however difficult they may feel you also have a greater sense of control. When you are faced with a stressful situation, try looking at it objectively and deciding how you can influence the situation by changing the circumstances or your own attitudes and behaviour. If you perceive the problem as worse than it really is you will subconsciously be sabotaging your ability to cope.

Assessing stressful events

Look at the list below and tick all the stressful events you have experienced over the last two years. Add up the score next to each source of stress you ticked, then look at the interpretation on page 104 to see how your experience of life events is likely to affect your health.

		Score
MAJOR STRESS	Death of a spouse	10
	Divorce	7
	Marital break-up	6
	Jail term	6
	Death of a close family member	6
	Personal injury or illness	5
	Marriage	5
	Loss of job	5
HIGH STRESS	Marital reconciliation	10
	Change in health of family member	7
	Pregnancy	6
	Sexual difficulties	6
	Gain of new family member	6
	Change to a different line of work	5
	Business readjustment	5
	Change in financial status	5
	Death of close friend	4
	Increased arguments with spouse	3

MODERATE STRESS

☐ Mortgage over £50,000	3
☐ Foreclosure of mortgage or loan	3
☐ Change in work responsibilities	3
☐ Son or daughter leaving home	3
☐ Trouble with in-laws	3
☐ Outstanding personal achievement	3
☐ Spouse begins or stops work	3
☐ Begin or end school/college	3
☐ Change in living conditions	3
☐ New year's resolutions	3
☐ Stopping smoking or drinking	3

LOW STRESS

☐ Trouble with boss	3
☐ Change in work hours or conditions	2
☐ Change of residence	2
☐ Change in recreation	2
☐ Change in social activities	2
☐ Mortgage or loan less than £50,000	2
☐ Change in sleeping habits	1
☐ Change in eating habits	1
☐ Holiday	1
☐ Christmas	1
☐ Minor run-ins with the law	1
☐ Other (add score of nearest item in list)	

SCORES

LESS THAN 10: Life has been kind to you over the last two years and not dealt you too many blows. The stress you have experienced is unlikely to damage your health.

11–20: Your life events score is acceptable but you need to look after your health. You've had a reasonable amount to deal with over the last two years, so take regular time out to relax.

21–30: Your life events score is high and the stress you are under is in danger of affecting your health. Another stressful event may just tip the balance.

OVER 30: Life has thrown so much at you over the last two years that your health is seriously at risk. Your reserves are running low and a minor event may prove to be the last straw. Stressed people who have been through one major life event after another are at increased risk of coronary heart disease, high blood pressure, stroke, mental illness and cancer. Consider seeking professional stress-counselling.

These figures are only intended to give you an idea of the amount of stress you are likely to be under. They are not meant to be exact, but help to remind you of all the events in your recent past that may have combined to affect your overall health.

Possible causes of stress

The possible causes of stress are varied and complex. Sometimes it is possible to determine a single cause and set about doing something about it but more often than not the causes of your stress are going to be interwoven. This chapter takes a close look at the following areas:

- Bereavement (page 106)
- Caring for the very young, infirm, elderly or disabled (page 109)
- Financial problems (page 111)
- Holidays (page 113)
- Major illness or injury (page 115)
- Menopause (page 117)
- Premenstrual syndrome (page 121)
- Shifting relationships (page123)
- Speaking in public (page 125)
- Work-related stress (page 127)

By filling in the questionnaire on the previous pages you will have discovered the main stressful areas in your life. Turn to any of those areas that are especially relevant and find how you can start removing the stress.

Bereavement

Sooner or later everyone will have to cope with bereavement. Whether it is the death of a parent, partner, child, family pet or close friend, the loss of a loved one is a devastating experience that affects your whole life and causes an enormous amount of stress. Everyone will react differently and every situation is different, but grief is a painful and isolating experience. Try not to be alone, however – even if you feel you want to shut yourself off from the outside world. Company is important at this difficult time. The support of family and friends is vital. You need to be able to talk about your feelings openly, without holding back. If someone asks how you feel, it is no use saying 'all right' if you feel absolutely awful. Take the opportunity to be honest about your emotions.

Anyone faced with death will feel unpleasant emotional symptoms such as shock, panic and helplessness at first. The facts take time to sink in, and feelings of unreality, such as, 'It can't be happening to me' or, 'This isn't real' are common. You may feel numb and find it difficult to cry – but it will help to let your emotions out and shed a few tears or even scream and shout. Time is your best friend: as the weeks and months pass, it gets easier to accept what has happened. You may feel guilty, that in some way you are to blame for what happened – again, this is a normal part of the grieving process. Later, you may feel angry at your loss, or jealous of others who have not had to go through what you have had to face. With time, you will start to accept what has happened and look to the future.

Everyone will eventually recover from the raw emotions, stresses and changes that result from a bereavement, but you will need to recover at your own pace and in your own time. Don't rush it as it is important to let the process run its natural course for you.

There are no right or wrong ways to grieve, and everyone copes differently. Sometimes, people who have suffered a bereavement slowly sink into depression. Depression can creep up on you, until you are overwhelmed with feelings of sadness, loneliness and despair.

When a loved one dies, it is also common to develop sleep problems. It can be difficult to get off to sleep, and when you do manage to nod off, you may find that your rest is disturbed by unusual dreams or that you wake earlier than normal. Sleep is one of nature's best healers, so it is important to get a good night's rest.

Self-help

- When you are coping with the stress of bereavement, it is important to voice your feelings and share them with others as this is a powerful part of the healing process.

- Thinking and talking about the person who has died will help keep their memory alive for you. To begin with this can be painful as it will bring raw emotions to the surface, but sharing your feelings is healthier than bottling them up.

- Try talking with a close friend or relative – someone who also knew the deceased person, as this will help you both.

- Some people find it easier to talk to someone removed from the situation, however, such as an uninvolved friend, doctor or a priest. You may even feel that professional bereavement counselling is what you need. Do whichever you feel most comfortable with.

- With time, you will be able to talk about the person with pleasure, remembering all the good times you shared. This is not 'dwelling in the past' or 'failing to get over it'. It is a healthy way of coping with your loss.

- When you can smile again, you will know you are well on the way to recovery.

- If you start feeling that things are getting on top of you, that you can no longer cope or that life is no longer worth living, it is important to seek help from your doctor. Depression is an important warning sign that the stress resulting from your bereavement is over-whelming and that you need professional help to come to terms with your loss.

- If it is your partner who has died, the bedroom will be associated with memories and it often helps to move into the spare room for a while or – even better – to stay with relatives or close friends.

- It can even help to phone someone and have a short conversation with a friend or relative before going to bed so you can voice any worries or thoughts that might otherwise stop you sleeping.

Caring for the very young, infirm, elderly or disabled

Caring for those who are very young, elderly, infirm or disabled is a rewarding task that can nevertheless be draining – physically and emotionally. It is important to help others maintain as much independence as possible but this will invariably lead to conflicting needs and demands, and a need for compromise that can be highly stressful.

Before you can care for others, you need to ensure you care for yourself. It is a common failing to ignore your own needs when those of others seem so much greater. You are not being selfish in taking the time for respite, however – you are ensuring that you – the carer of those you love – remain physically and emotionally equal to the task. Ask yourself what would happen if your health or strength were to fail too. Where would everyone be then?

Self-help

- Take regular breaks from stressful situations.

- If you are caring for someone who is dependent night and day, make sure you have some nights off to allow you to sleep through.

- If caring for someone at home, seek advice to ensure you are receiving all the financial benefits to which you and the person you are caring for are entitled.

- Go out socially at least once a week – even if it is only window shopping or for a stroll with a friend.

- Talk to other family members about how you feel and how you are coping – don't bottle your emotions up.

- If you need extra help, don't be afraid to ask for it. Practise your assertiveness skills. You may even find that friends and family have been holding back from offering to help for fear they may offend you.

- Keep up an outside hobby or interest such as gardening, writing to a penpal or researching a topic that interests you in the local library.

- Keep active – physical fitness is important. Take steps to lose any excess weight and consider joining a yoga class for relaxation, a swimming class for fitness or perhaps a rambling club to meet new people. If the person you care for needs constant supervision, ask friends, relatives, neighbours or self-help/charity groups to help organize a rota that gives you regular time off each week for an outside activity.

- When stress builds up, use visualization, meditation, breathing exercises or a relaxation technique to help you regain control.

Financial problems

Money worries are frequently present in most families. Even people who seem to be doing well often have a shaky financial foundation with large overheads, an overdraft and a bank manager who, although outwardly friendly and accommodating, may have to change his priorities at short notice to protect his bank's investors.

No matter how tight or flush your finances, unexpected expenses can cause stress if you have not made suitable plans to cope with monetary changes: either in outgoings or in income.

Self-help

- Record where your money comes from and where it goes to in up-to-date household accounts – keep everything together in one filing drawer, desk or concertina file so that everything is immediately at hand.

- If economies have to be made, it is surprisingly easy to pull in your horns and reduce outgoings with a concerted economy drive.

- Keep track of when bills have to be paid – especially credit card bills. Missing a payment or paying late attracts stiff financial penalties.

- Talk to the financial advisor at your bank to see what services are available and how much they cost – it often pays to take out a small overdraft or loan to pay off credit cards balances as the annual interest rate is usually much less.

- Set yourself a weekly or monthly budget, and stick to it. If the budget is tight, aim to balance income and outgoings – don't allow small deficits to start accumulating at the end of each month.

- Try to put aside a certain amount of money each month as savings – no matter how small – in a savings account where you can access it fairly quickly if necessary.

- Once you have sufficient cash built up in an account for emergencies, seek independent financial planning about how to build up further 'safe' nest eggs according to the amount of risk you are prepared to take.

- Seek independent advice on financial planning services such as insurance, pensions and planning for redundancy or critical illness. Think hard about taking on any new financial commitments, however – no matter how good the deal seems. Remember that nothing comes free – every deal is intended to make money, somewhere, for someone else.

- Everyone should ensure they have made a will. Although there is no legal obligation to do so, the lack of one will result in major stress and possible money problems for surviving members of your family should you die. Look upon your will as your family's insurance for the future and your right to ensure your wishes are carried out after your death. Having made a will, it is equally important to keep it up-to-date, especially if financial circumstances change and this could have implications for inheritance tax.

Holidays

Holidays feature surprisingly high on most people's list of major stresses. While poring over brochures and dreaming of exotic destinations can aid your visualization skills, it is easy to invest so much emotional energy in your holiday that it inevitably turns into an anticlimax. Try to keep a sense of realism on your side at all times. Many people would have a more pleasant and relaxing time if they stayed at home for a change.

Common causes of holiday stress

- Preparation
- Packing – deciding what to take and fitting it into available space
- Organizing passports, tickets, insurance, immunizations
- Additional unexpected costs
- Sorting out what to do with pets and dependent relatives
- Travelling with small children
- Motion sickness
- Queues, delays and overbookings at the airport
- Destination not what was expected
- Overcrowded resorts and excessive noise
- Running round doing and seeing too much until you are exhausted
- Culture shock

- Poor weather
- Traveller's illnesses, especially vomiting and diarrhoea
- Indigestion from foods you are not used to
- Sunburn and insect bites/stings
- Coming home to find a pipe has burst or you have been burgled
- Returning to work with an overflowing in-tray and everyone demanding large chunks of your time
- Next month's credit card bill: you overspent or were caught out by credit-card fraud

Why did you ever go away in the first place?

By staying at home on holiday, you can:

- Lie in and have a leisurely breakfast
- Read the paper from cover to cover for a change
- Read that book you keep meaning to get around to
- Spend a little of the money you've saved in not going away on having a few good meals in a local restaurant, going to the cinema/theatre, buying a barbecue for fun evenings on the patio
- Spend time exploring local beauty spots and tourist attractions you would otherwise never get around to seeing
- Invite friends around for a dinner or drinks party
- Spend more quality time with your family

Major illness or injury

Serious illness either in yourself or those you are close to is a powerful cause of stress, especially when there is uncertainty. Some illnesses and accidents have temporary effects from which, although it may be touch and go to begin with, a full recovery is usually made. This allows you to achieve a sense of closure, the stress recedes and you can carry on with life much as before. When an illness or injury has long-term consequences, however, your life will inevitably change from what it was. Major illness or injury can trigger many different causes of stress such as:

- Worrying about the significance of various symptoms
- Having to endure a series of tests and then await results
- Having to face a serious diagnosis
- Coping with pain, immobility, changes in certain bodily functions or coping with treatments that may have unpleasant side effects
- Having to face surgery and/or fear of disfigurement
- Frustration at infirmity
- Anger – feelings of 'why me?' or 'why us?'
- Guilt or remorse – feelings of 'if only'
- Uncertainty and fear about the future
- Worry about how loved ones will cope
- Fear that things are being kept from you or fear of loss of control
- Coming to terms with your own mortality

After a traumatic event, it is common to suffer from post-traumatic stress disorder in which you may experience anxiety, flashbacks, panic attacks, difficulty sleeping, depression, avoiding anything linked with the event, and feelings of guilt, remorse, anger or even shame. Don't bottle up your emotions – let them out. Talk about your feelings and once you have made a good recovery, try to get back to normal as soon as possible within the limits of your condition.

Self-help

- It is no good dwelling on what might have been or what you could have done differently. The best way to fight any illness is to face it head on, steel yourself for what lies ahead and make plans about the best way to cope. Negative thinking will drag you down and slow the healing process.

- When feeling stressed by illness or pain, it can help to practise a breathing exercise, a relaxation technique or to visualize yourself fighting the illness and becoming well again.

- The power of mind over body is phenomenal, and positive thinking will reduce pain, improve the body's ability to heal itself and help you cope.

- If you feel you need extra help, don't be afraid to ask for it. Counselling is especially important if you are suffering the effects of post-traumatic stress, and your doctor can refer you if necessary.

Menopause

The menopause is often called the 'change of life', and as we have already seen, change is one of the most common causes of stress. The word *menopause* literally means the time when your last period stops. This normally occurs between the ages of 45 and 55, the average being 51 years. Some lifestyle factors can bring on your menopause earlier than otherwise expected. Heavy smokers reach the menopause an average of two years earlier than a non-smoker. Excess alcohol also poisons egg-follicle cells to trigger an earlier menopause. High levels of stress also affect hormone balance and can trigger the menopause significantly earlier than expected – so the menopause can both result from excess stress and contribute to increased stress levels. Many women find that sex feels different after the menopause, and as oestrogen levels fall, one in five experience a profound loss of interest in sex. This is another powerful cause (and effect) of stress.

Although the menopause is dated from the last period, it really starts five to ten years before – during a woman's early to mid-forties – when the number of eggs remaining in the ovaries decreases and levels of the female hormone oestrogen naturally start to fall. When levels eventually become too low to control the monthly cycle, menstruation will stop. Some women quickly adapt to lower levels of oestrogen and notice few – if any – problems. Others find it harder to lose their oestrogen and experience unpleasant symptoms that last from one to five years – and occasionally longer.

Women who are experiencing a lot of stress seem more likely to suffer distressing symptoms around the time of the menopause than those with a less demanding lifestyle. Usually the adrenal glands help to smooth out the effects of falling oestrogen levels by producing extra amounts of other sex hormones that can be converted into oestrogen. If you have been under long-term stress, however, the adrenal glands are already working flat out making extra stress hormones such as adrenaline, noradrenaline and cortisol, and have no extra reserves to boost oestrogen levels to even out hormonal fluctuations at this time.

Preparing for the menopause

Every woman will eventually approach the menopause. To help make your passage through these changes easier there are a number of steps you can take before your first symptoms start:

- Follow a healthy diet that is low in fat and contains plenty of fresh fruit, vegetables, salad-stuff and unrefined, complex carbohydrates.

- Start increasing the amount of exercise you take to improve your fitness level.

- Try to lose any excess weight.

- If you smoke, make a major effort to stop.

- Keep your alcohol limit to within the recommended safe maximum for women of no more than two or three drinks a day and try to have at least one alcohol-free day per week.

- Don't let yourself be overburdened with tasks – learn to say 'no' and mean it so that people don't put upon you.
- Find time for relaxation and quiet, at least half an hour per day – soaking in an aromatherapy bath surrounded with flickering candle-light is a great way to end the day, for example.
- Keep your mind active and your spirits up with a new hobby such as learning a foreign language, taking painting lessons or joining a rambling club.

Self-help

- Eat plants rich in natural oestrogen-like plant hormones, such as soya-bean products, celery, fennel, chinese leaves and other green or yellow vegetables.
- Cut back on sugar, salt, tea, coffee and caffeinated fizzy drinks.
- If suffering from hot flushes, avoid spicy foods and convenience foods.
- Avoid alcohol and smoking cigarettes, which lower oestrogen levels further.
- Try taking evening primrose oil (3000 mg) per day for at least three months to see if it helps.
- If suffering from hot flushes, vaginal dryness, night sweats of anxiety, Siberian ginseng often helps.
- Consult a homeopath for a remedy that matches your symptoms (see page 180).

- Aromatherapy essential oils have powerful effects on your moods. Many are also oestrogenic when absorbed from the skin into your circulation and can help to improve menopausal symptoms. Always use aromatherapy oils in a diluted form by adding a maximum of 5 drops to each 10 ml of carrier oil (almond or grapeseed, for example). This is because some neat oils can cause skin irritation. Diluted oils may be massaged into your skin, added to bath water or diffused into the air to scent your room. Do not use during pregnancy except under advice from a qualified aromatherapist. Aromatherapy oils that help relieve oestrogen-withdrawal symptoms such as hot flushes, sweating and vaginal dryness include camomile, clary sage, cypress, fennel, geranium, grapefruit, lemon, lime, rose and sage.

- St John's wort is effective in lifting mild to moderate depression. One trial showed that *hypericum* plus black cohosh was effective in treating 78 per cent of women with hot flushes and other menopausal problems within two to four weeks.

- Soya extracts have been shown to help reduce menopausal symptoms such as hot flushes and night sweats.

- Wild yam (*Dioscorea villosa*) is rich in hormone building-blocks from which progesterone can be synthesized in the laboratory. The body cannot carry out this conversion itself, but wild yam does seem to have some useful progestogenic actions that many women find helpful at the menopause.

Premenstrual syndrome

Premenstrual Syndrome (PMS) is a common and distressing problem
that affects at least three-quarters of menstruating women. Half have
significant symptoms, and for one in 20, these are incapacitating, neces-
sitating regular days off work. PMS is associated with a variety of
symptoms that come on in the 14 days before a period is due and
disappear soon after bleeding starts. Problems include headache,
backache, bloating, cyclical breast pain, tiredness and food cravings.
Many emotional symptoms also occur such as anxiety, poor concentration, irritability, weepiness, mood swings, low sex drive and depression.
In some cases, PMS is so bad the personality of the sufferer changes.
PMS is therefore well recognized as a stressful event for many women
and one that, unfortunately, can recur every few weeks. In extreme
cases, it may affect a woman as long as two weeks out of every four.

Self-help

- Eat little and often – be a grazer rather than a gorger.

- Eat a low-fat carbohydrate snack (for example, crispbreads, digestive
  biscuits, toast, rice cakes) every three hours, starting as soon as you
  wake. This helps maintain blood glucose levels.

- Eat oily fish three times a week (sardines, herrings, pilchards,
  salmon, mackerel, trout) for the essential fatty acids they contain.

- Eat at least five portions of fruit and vegetables per day, especially green leafy vegetables for their vitamin, mineral, fibre and antioxidant content.

- Take evening primrose oil, which contains hormone building-blocks that can even out imbalances. You will need to take up to 3000 mg a day for at least three months before an effect may be noticed.

- Follow a healthy, organic, wholefood diet with low intakes of salt, additives, table sugar, monosodium glutamate, caffeine and alcohol.

- Take a vitamin and mineral supplement especially designed for women with PMS, which includes B-group vitamins (100 mg per day) and magnesium (300–500 mg per day).

- Take regular exercise – this helps to burn off excess adrenaline levels and is therefore helpful for reducing PMS symptoms in the long term.

- Consult a homeopath for a remedy that matches your symptoms (see page 180).

- The aromatherapy essential oils of geranium and rosemary can relieve water retention. Add a few drops to a hankie for inhalation, or dilute with a carrier oil and use in the bath or for an abdominal massage (do not use during pregnancy).

- Stimulation of the bladder and kidney meridians by acupuncture is often successful in banishing excess fluid.

- Manipulation of the feet at points corresponding to the kidneys, bladder and lymphatic areas using reflexology may help.

Shifting relationships

Many causes of stress come from emotions triggered by your close inter-
actions with your immediate family. Have a look at this list and tick
those that have previously been a cause of stress in your life or which
are affecting you now.

- [ ] Committing to a partner either through engagement, living
  together or marriage

- [ ] Becoming a parent

- [ ] Family rows with parents, in-laws or young children

- [ ] Problems with adolescents

- [ ] Problems with step families

- [ ] Children leaving home

- [ ] Separation and/or divorce

- [ ] Extra-marital affairs

- [ ] Mid-life crisis and the need to be free from others to 'find yourself'

The advertising stereotype of happy smiling families is only a small
snapshot on reality; although we are social animals, living closely with
others causes frequent ups and downs. Everyone has their own way of
doing things and these may sometimes conflict with those around us.
One of the main causes of family problems is lack of communication.
Most families would benefit from talking to each other more in a direct,

open and honest way. One of the biggest culprits in this respect is the television – after a hard day at work or school, it is easier to sit in front of the box and be entertained than to talk to the rest of the family and find out what has happened in their world while you were away.

Self-help

- If family dynamics are causing you stress, try to work out what the problems are and how many can be addressed by sitting down together and talking things through.

- A discussion aimed at addressing the root causes of relationship stresses needs to be frank and open, not hidden behind gestures, inferences, veiled comments, jokes or put-downs.

- It is important to be clear and positive in what you are saying, so think about what you want to say beforehand and how you are going to say it.

- Don't express your feelings as a criticism or blame; use 'I' language – rather than saying, 'You ...', say, 'I would prefer it if ...'.

- Stick to the point and try not to get sidetracked until the issue has been resolved.

- Don't bottle up your emotions – express your feelings and don't be afraid to cry. Crying is a great reliever of stress. It is important to have someone close you can talk to or confide in – but it must be someone you trust, such as a close family member or an old friend. If you lack this sort of support, remember that the Samaritans are always on the end of the phone to listen – just call 08457 909090.

Speaking in public

It is surprising how many people are filled with panic at the thought of speaking in public. Yet many people have to do this as part of their work and quickly come to realize there is no great mystery about the ability to do so, it just comes down to practice. Think about some of the presenters you have watched on TV, thinking, 'I could do better than that.' Well, you can. Public speaking is an art that is easily learned. Although some personality types such as the forceful and the extrovert will find it easier than others, practice will make perfect every time.

Self-help

- First of all, believe in yourself: you *can* do it.

- Prepare in advance by finding out who your audience is, what they want to hear from you, why you need to speak to them and how best to get your message across.

- Practise in advance: prepare notes on small index cards and use these to talk out loud in the privacy of your bedroom, bathroom, a field, your garden – wherever you won't be overheard.

- Use visualization exercises to imagine yourself giving the talk perfectly, exactly as you have practised (see page 193).

- Wear clothes that are appropriately smart and comfortable.

- Learn a breathing exercise to help calm you on the day. Also, for ten seconds before you start, take a deep, long, slow breath in through your nose, then slowly release it through your mouth. Use Rescue Remedy flower essence as necessary.

- Smile!
- Don't start until you feel ready. Take your time. Similarly, feel comfortable with pausing to collect your thoughts during your talk. If you make a mistake, don't panic. Pause, then start again.
- Greet the audience as a warm-up and to get the feel for your voice – don't forget to speak up.
- Make eye-contact with your audience while speaking, sweeping your gaze around to all corners so no one feels excluded.
- Don't fiddle, click a pen or jingle coins in your pocket.
- Smile while talking and animate your face – look interested in what you are saying.
- Use light humour to get the audience on your side, but be careful only to poke fun at yourself – not at others.
- Be brief and to the point. Try to stick to three main messages and get your most important point across first. It often helps to:

    1. Say what you are going to say.

    2. Say it.

    3. Then say what you have said.

- Get your audience to do some of the work: don't be afraid to ask questions.

Work-related stress

Most people spend the major part of their waking life at work, and more often than not you are identified with the type of work you do. People will say, for example, he is an architect, she is a professor of anthropology, he is an electrician, she is unemployed. Your work goes a long way towards denoting your status in life, and it is common practice for social introductions to include a statement or questions about what someone does for a living. As well as paying the bills, work should be a valuable source of satisfaction and of positive pressure. All too often, however, it becomes a source of negative stress.

What happens to you at work is important to your health and well-being. When you lose your job, it means far more than just losing a source of income; it can feel like a judgement on your lack of worth and lead to low self-image, a feeling of helplessness, increased fatalism and loss of essential contact with other people.

Job stress can undermine your sense of personal worth and dignity. Different administrative styles can stir up different kinds of unconscious conflicts within each member of a group. Different jobs are carried out by different types of worker – engineer, secretary, executive or printer – yet everyone expects to gain satisfaction from the particular job they perform. Nowadays, workers are demanding an increasing degree of fulfilment as human beings.

Stress and the working woman

The number of women working outside the home has more than doubled over the last 25 years. Many women work because of economic necessity, but increasing numbers work out of choice. Although the so-called glass barriers that make it difficult for women to advance in certain careers do still exist, women frequently now achieve senior posts as captains of industry, eminent scholars or capable politicians. Despite these achievements, women often pay an additional price for their success over and above that paid by male colleagues. For example, there is the familiar conflict between pursuing a career and rearing a family. Some studies suggest that men look on their home environment as a support system while women may see it more as a burden. As a result, women executives are far less likely to give their home life a high priority compared with their male peers and are twice as likely to be single or divorced. This is not surprising given that many women finish a full day's work at the office and are then still expected to do more than their fair share of cooking and household chores on arriving home.

Many women cope with the stress they feel due to the pressure of conflicting home and work demands through excessive eating, smoking, drinking and medication, all of which damage their health further and drain them of vitality. The nurturing role is not only burdensome in itself, but the conflict between playing the traditional role and developing an independent career outside the home is even more exhausting. Women are constantly at odds with themselves trying to perform both roles.

In addition to carrying the dual load, women also have to put up with physiological disadvantages. Many women suffer from premenstrual syndrome, which may affect the quality of their work and makes them more irritable and accident-prone, and more likely to make rash decisions (see page 121). In addition, women reaching the end of their fertile life may also develop troublesome menopausal symptoms.

What causes you stress at work?

Consider the following questions and see if any apply to your situation.

- Have you recently lost your job?
- Have you recently changed your job?
- Have you just taken on an additional new job?
- Have changes at work resulted in increased demands upon you?
- Have you recently been promoted?
- Have the immediate colleagues you work with changed?
- Have you recently had a new boss?
- Have you recently been placed in charge of new people yourself?
- Is your role and power base ambiguous?
- Are your skills underused?
- Do you feel overloaded with work?
- Are relationships at work a source of stress?
- Do you find using office technology a source of stress?

- Are you having to cope with study for work-related exams?
- Is the threat of redundancy hanging over your head?
- Do you find commuting and experiences of road rage stressful?

Unrealistic aims may be set, by yourself or your boss; work facilities may be inadequate; you may experience role conflicts with other people in the office. Just one of these major challenges will raise the pressure you are under, but small things can add up over time as well, such as:

- numerous deadlines – lack of feedback or appreciation from the top for how well you are doing – responsibility without adequate authority – unclear goals – boss with an abrasive or weak leadership style – lack of communication about serious problems in the company – lack of leadership in times of crisis – feeling trapped in an unsatisfying job.

And that's not all. Physical and psychological environment stressors can also come into play to make your work life stressful:

- unsuitable chairs that cannot be individually ergonomically adjusted – desk too high or too low – lack of personal work space – undue clutter or lack of storage/filing space – noisy surroundings – poor lighting – VDU screen glare – lack of access to natural light – having to stand, walk or bend all day – office politics, whether you are actively involved in them or not – sarcastic remarks or put-downs from colleagues – malicious office gossip – bullying and racial, ageist or sexual harassment – having to work in isolation – having to work in an overcrowded environment – having to work in an inhospitable physical environment (for example, having to wear bulky protective clothing or deep-sea diving equipment; having to work in sterile conditions or with toxins) – having to work in shifts.

Self-help

Having looked at the lists above and worked out some of the sources of your work-related stress, it will help to plan constructive ways round the major problems. Study the following coping strategies and put a tick next to those you believe you already practise effectively, and a cross by those where you need to improve your skills.

- Time management
- Setting sensible priorities
- Planning skills
- Delegation
- Keeping to a sensible workload
- Communication
- Pacing yourself – taking time out for meals and teabreaks will energize you
- Sticking to your contracted hours more closely and leaving for home at a sensible hour
- Improved communication within the company

Keeping a stress diary

Keeping a detailed diary will help you assess more immediate events in your life so that you can identify your main causes of stress and pinpoint any patterns. It will also help to show how effective your responses to stress are, and help you plan alternative strategies to avoid similar feelings of stress in the future.

Be honest with yourself and record the events from a dispassion-ate point of view. Keep the diary with you at all times, and try to fill it in after each event. Don't leave it until the end of the day – by then you will not be able to accurately record how you felt.

When you have completed a week check the material recorded in the diary. It will provide you with several useful pieces of information to help you plan the next steps in your stress-busting campaign.

- Which situations caused you most stress, and why?
- Are the main sources of your feelings of stress internal or external?
- Which feelings of stress were due to change or things imposed on you, and how much control are you able to exert over them?
- How do you perceive the situations that make you feel most stressed?
- What do you use as safety valves?
- Were your responses appropriate?
- Could you have reacted differently, in a more constructive way?

SAMPLE DIARY ENTRY – FRIDAY

TIME	SITUATION	FEELINGS	NEGATIVE RESPONSE	POSSIBLE CORRECTIVE ACTIONS
08.45	Stuck in traffic	Frustrated – afraid will be late for work again	Tried listening to Classic FM	Leave home earlier in future.
09.10	Late for work again – boss threatened a written warning	Dreadfully worried and afraid this will affect promotion prospects	Over-ate at break-time –a doughnut and a creambun – yuk!	Apologize firmly to boss and promise it will not happen again. Don't go to canteen – take fruit to work instead.
10.00	Unpleasant phone-call from an irate customer	Upset, angry. It wasn't my fault the wrong goods were sent	Burst into tears – too much pressure	Attend a course on assertiveness and self-esteem for women.
17.30	Shopped in crowded supermarket with long queues	Frustrated, hot and snappy with check-out girl for being so slow	Cut shopping short – went home without several vital items	Go for a run to burn off effects of stress hormones. Shop when supermarket quieter. Look into having fruit and veg delivered by local organic farming co-op.
19.00	Picked row with spouse for coming into house with dirty, muddy shoes	Even more upset – no one appreciates all I do for them	Phoned friend for a long moan. Cracked open a bottle of wine and drank most of it myself – husband stormed out to the pub	Make up with spouse – explain we've both had a stressful day and are taking it out on our nearest and dearest. Drive to a quiet country pub for a relaxing evening and a quiet, candle-lit meal for two (forgot to buy the steaks for supper anyway!). Watch alcohol intake – stick to spritzers.

3 EAT WISELY

A nutritious, well-balanced diet makes for a healthy body that is vibrant
with energy. When you are under stress and juggling too many things in
your life, it is easy to adopt an unhealthy diet and lifestyle. The old
saying, 'you are what you eat' is increasingly known to be true. Every
building-block in your body is ultimately derived from your food, which
must provide all the vitamins, minerals, fibre, essential fatty acids,
protein and energy needed for optimum health. Chinese medicine
teaches that poor eating habits negatively affect physical, mental and
spiritual health while a good diet increases feelings of well-being and
energy.

Caffeine

Caffeine has a chemical effect in your body that mimics the adrenaline
stress response. A person weighing 11 stone (70 kg) who drinks more
than six caffeine-containing drinks per day (for example, six cups of
coffee) can easily develop caffeine poisoning, whose symptoms are restlessness, irritability, headache, insomnia and tiredness. It is therefore a
good idea to make sure your intake does not go up at times of stress.
Limit coffee and other caffeinated drinks to three cups a day or switch

to decaffeinated brands. Herbal or fruit teas are an excellent soothing alternative. Although tea contains some caffeine, it is also rich in flavonoids – the chemicals known to give red wine its beneficial properties. Research suggests that drinking four cups of tea a day may halve your risk of a heart attack. When under stress, it is therefore worth switching from drinking coffee to drinking tea. Green tea may be more beneficial than black, fermented tea.

Salt

Table salt is commonly used to flavour food, and excess has been linked with an increased risk of high blood pressure. This sensitivity seems to be dependent on the genes you have inherited and affects around one in two people. The effects of stress will magnify this response, so if you are under excess pressure it is worth cutting back on your salt intake.

Ideally, you should take no more than 4–6 g salt a day. The average intake is 6 g, however, with some people eating as much as 12 g salt daily. Unfortunately, around three-quarters of dietary salt is hidden in processed foods such as tinned products, ready-prepared meals, biscuits, cakes, meat products and breakfast cereals.

Cut down on salt gradually and season your food with spices, black pepper and herbs instead – that way, you won't miss it.

When checking labels, those giving salt content as sodium need to be multiplied by 2.5 to give true salt content: for example, a serving of soup containing 0.4 g sodium contains 1 g salt.

The importance of breakfast

Eating a healthy breakfast gets you off to a good start for the day. Forget bacon and eggs, however – the best power breakfast contains cereal, fruit and skimmed or semi-skimmed milk. Not only can a low-fat, high-carbohydrate breakfast improve your physical performance during the day, but new research shows that a cereal breakfast acts as a stress-buster for adults. Those who regularly eat cereals first thing in the morning were found to be less depressed, less emotionally distressed and to have lower stress levels than those not eating breakfast. Eating a cereal breakfast has also been found to improve your mood and memory – especially for those over the age of 60 years. It increases the speed at which new information can be recalled, and improves concentration and mental performance. As a result, it will help you work more effectively during the morning and encourage a positive mood so you cope better with situations that could otherwise lead to stress.

Regularly eating a cereal breakfast has also been shown to help protect against the common cold. Researchers found that only around one in six of those eating a cereal breakfast every day developed a cold over the ten-week study, compared with one in three of those who ate a cereal breakfast less than once a week. Whether this is due to the cereal, the fortified vitamins and minerals it contains or even the milk that accompanies it is uncertain.

The food pyramid

One of the most popular ways of depicting healthy eating is in the form of the food pyramid. At the base of the pyramid are the complex carbohydrates, of which you need to eat around 5–11 portions daily. Next up are the fruit and vegetable group, of which you need to eat 5–9 portions a day. As a source of protein animal and dairy products should be limited to 2–3 portions a day, while at the top of the pyramid are the fats, oils, sugars and sweets, which you should only eat infrequently.

Carbohydrate

Dietary carbohydrates provide your main source of energy and should ideally provide at least half your daily energy intake. This should mostly be in the form of complex, unrefined carbohydrates such as wholegrain cereals, brown rice, wholemeal bread, wholewheat pasta and jacket potatoes, since these contain additional valuable nutrients such as vitamins, trace elements and dietary fibre.

Some forms of carbohydrate cause large blood-sugar swings and are one of the internal triggers for the adrenaline stress response when blood-sugar levels rebound too low.

The way in which different foods make your blood-sugar levels rise is known as their glycaemic index (GI). For general health – and especially when you are under pressure – it is best to eat foods with a low to moderate GI, and to combine foods with a high GI with those that have a lower GI to help even out fluctuations in blood-sugar levels.

Another benefit of eating complex carbohydrates is that they trigger the release of a brain chemical, serotonin, which helps to lift your mood and also controls your desire for food. By eating a high-carbohydrate diet, you will feel full quicker and eat less food overall. You are also less likely to suffer from low moods. Low levels of serotonin have been linked with overeating and carbohydrate cravings. Dietary carbohydrate also boosts your metabolic rate, speeds up the rate at which you burn excess energy, and makes you feel more energized.

Fruit and vegetables

Fruit and vegetables – including nuts, seeds, pulses and wholegrains – are a rich source of water, carbohydrate, proteins, vitamins, minerals, fibre, essential fatty acids and at least 20 non-nutrient substances, known as phytochemicals, which help to protect our health and immunity. Many of these substances are powerful antioxidants (see page 145) that help to boost immune function and protect against a variety of conditions, including some cancers.

Aim to eat at least a pound (454 g) in weight of fruit, vegetables or salad-stuff per day, not counting potatoes. This works out at around five servings. This may seem like a lot but is fairly easy to do – for example, the following adds up to a healthy total of seven servings:

- fresh orange juice with breakfast
- banana mid-morning
- a large salad with lunch

- an apple mid-afternoon
- broccoli and sweetcorn with dinner
- fresh fruit salad for dessert.

Protein

Proteins are made up of building-blocks called amino acids. When you eat protein, it is digested down into individual amino acids which are then recombined to make the more than 50,000 different proteins that are needed to keep the body working properly. Twenty amino acids are important for human health. Of these, ten cannot be synthesized in the body in amounts needed by the metabolism and must therefore come from the diet. These are known as the nutritionally essential amino acids. Dietary protein can be divided into two groups:

- First-class proteins contain significant quantities of the essential amino acids, for example animal meat, fish, eggs, dairy products.
- Second-class proteins contain some of the essential amino acids but not all, for example vegetables, rice, beans, nuts.

Second-class proteins need to be mixed and matched by eating as wide a variety of foods as possible.

The average adult male needs to obtain around 56 g protein a day from his food. Protein deficiency is uncommon in the West, where most people obtain 80–90g protein a day from their food, with around a third of this coming from meat or meat products.

Dietary fats

A certain amount of fat is important for health and is needed for healthy cell membranes and nerve function, and to provide building-blocks to maintain hormone balance. It is estimated that as many as one in three heart attacks are due to an unhealthy diet with too much fat and not enough starchy foods or fruit and vegetables. Fats are the richest dietary source of energy and most people eat too much. Ideally, fats should provide no more than 30 per cent of your daily energy intake.

Essential fatty acids

There are many different sorts of fats in the diet and some, known as essential fatty acids (EFAs), are vital for health. These cannot be made in the body and must therefore come from your food. EFAs are found in nuts, seeds, green leafy vegetables, oily fish and wholegrains, or by taking supplements such as evening primrose and omega-3 fish oils. It is estimated that as many as eight out of ten people do not get enough EFAs from their diet. In addition, metabolic pathways involved in the metabolism of EFAs can be blocked by excess intakes of saturated fat, sugar and alcohol, lack of vitamins and minerals, smoking cigarettes or being under excess stress.

For a healthy fat intake, especially when you are under stress:

- Concentrate on eating beneficial fats such as olive, rapeseed, walnut, fish and evening primrose oils.

- Avoid obviously fatty foods.
- Cut back on beefburgers, sausages, pies, pizza, crisps, chips, pastries, cakes, doughnuts, chocolate and cream.
- Trim excess fat from meat and only use lean cuts.
- Eat chicken in preference to fatty meats such as pork.
- Grill food rather than frying to help fat drain away.
- Soak up excess fat from cooked foods using kitchen paper.
- Eat baked potatoes rather than roasted or chipped.
- Have several vegetarian meals, which include pulses and beans for protein, each week.
- Switch to reduced-fat versions of mayonnaise, salad dressing, cheese, milk and yoghurt.
- Eat red meat only once or twice a week and have more vegetarian meals instead.
- Try to reduce your intake of margarines and processed foods.

Fibre

Dietary fibre – or roughage – refers to the indigestible parts of plants. There are two main types of dietary fibre: soluble and insoluble. Soluble fibre is important in the stomach and upper intestines, where it slows digestion and absorption to ensure blood sugar and fat rise relatively slowly so that the metabolism can handle nutrient fluctuations more easily.

Insoluble fibre is most important in the large bowel. It bulks up the faeces, absorbs water and toxins and hastens stool excretion.

A high-fibre diet helps to keep your bowel function healthy during times of stress and can frequently help to reduce symptoms of irritable bowel syndrome, especially constipation.

It is important to eat as many different sources of fibre as possible and good sources include bran, dried apricots, peas, prunes, brown rice, and wholemeal pasta and bread. New research suggests that bowel bacteria quickly adapt to the types of roughage in your diet. If you mainly eat fibre of one type (for example, a bran supplement) your bowel bacteria will respond within a week or two by increasing their output of enzymes needed to ferment this. The fibre reaching your colon will then be broken down more quickly so that you lose much of the benefit gained.

Ideally, everyone needs to eat at least 30 g fibre per day. The easiest way to increase the amount of fibre in your diet is to eat more unrefined complex carbohydrates in foods such as wholemeal bread, cereals, nuts, grains, root vegetables and fruits. Bran-containing breakfast cereals provide one of the highest concentrations of dietary fibre.

Vitamins

Vitamins are naturally occurring organic substances that are essential for life, although they are only needed in minute amounts. Vitamins cannot be synthesized in the body in enough quantity to meet your needs and must therefore come from your food. Most vitamins work by boosting the rate at which important metabolic reactions occur in your cells such as those involved in the digestion of foods, converting fats and carbohydrates into energy, cell growth and division, overcoming stress reactions and mopping up harmful by-products of metabolism such as free radicals.

Some vitamins and minerals, for example vitamin C and the vitamin B complex, are quickly used up during stress reactions. Vitamin B is further depleted by the metabolism of alcohol and sugary foods, which are often resorted to in difficult times. As vitamin B deficiency in itself can lead to symptoms of anxiety and irritability, a vicious circle is set up that may make anxiety and irritability worse.

Cereals are a rich source of vitamin B1 (thiamine), which has a beneficial effect on mood, so you feel more calm, agreeable, clear-headed, elated and energetic. People with low levels of thiamine are less likely to feel composed or self-confident and more likely to suffer from depression than those with higher levels.

Other foods rich in vitamin B1 that will help to produce a stress-busting effect are: brewer's yeast and yeast extract, brown rice, wheatgerm and wheat bran, wholegrain bread and cereals, oatmeal and oatflakes, soya flour, pasta, meat, seafood, pulses and nuts.

Minerals

Minerals are inorganic elements, some of which are metals, that are also essential for healthy metabolism. Those needed in amounts of less than 100 mg are often referred to as trace elements. Minerals and trace elements can only come from your diet and depend on the quality of soil on which produce is grown or grazed. Minerals have a number of functions:

- Structural, for example, calcium, magnesium and phosphate, which strengthen bones and teeth.
- Maintaining normal cell function, for example, sodium, potassium, calcium.
- Co-factor for important enzymes, for example, copper, iron, magnesium, manganese, molybdenum, selenium, zinc.
- Involved in oxygen transport, for example, iron.
- Hormone function, for example, chromium, iodine.
- Antioxidant, for example, selenium, manganese.

Some trace elements, such as nickel, tin and vanadium are known to be essential for normal growth in only tiny amounts, although their exact roles are not yet fully understood.

Vitamin and mineral supplements

During times of stress, your need for antioxidant vitamins and minerals, and those involved in energy-producing reactions goes up. B-group vitamins in particular are depleted during times of stress and when drinking excess alcohol.

It is estimated that only one in ten people get all the vitamins, minerals and essential fatty acids they need from their foods. Although diet should always come first, it is important to ensure a good intake of vitamins and minerals when you are under excess pressure. It is therefore worth taking a good multi-nutrient supplement providing around 100 per cent of the recommended daily amount (RDA) of as many vitamins and minerals as possible. Evening primrose oil (1,000 mg daily) will also help to ensure a good intake of essential fatty acids.

Coenzyme Q10 is a vitamin-like substance important for the release of energy in cells. It is also believed to keep blood-vessel walls healthy and to regulate blood pressure. Supplements containing coenzyme Q10 improve heart muscle function and can reduce high blood pressure. If you are under stress, lacking in energy or have high blood pressure, coenzyme Q10 may be beneficial.

Antioxidants

Antioxidants are protective substances that patrol the body, mopping up harmful by-products of metabolism, stress and disease known as free radicals. The most important dietary antioxidants are vitamins A (and betacarotene), C and E, selenium, riboflavin, copper and manganese.

A free radical is an unstable molecular fragment that carries a minute, negative electrical charge in the form of a spare electron. It tries to lose this charge by colliding with other molecules and cell structures in a process known as oxidation. Oxidation usually triggers a harmful chain reaction in which electrons are passed from one molecule to another with damaging results. Free radicals are produced by:

- Metabolism in body cells, especially during times of stress
- Muscles during exercise
- Smoking cigarettes
- Drinking excessive amounts of alcohol
- Exposure to environmental pollutants
- Exposure to x-rays
- Exposure to UVA sunlight, especially if sunburned
- Taking some drugs – especially antibiotics or paracetamol

Body proteins, fats, cell membranes and genetic material (DNA) are constantly under attack from free radicals, with each cell undergoing an estimated 10,000 free radical oxidations per day. These collisions and chain reactions have been linked with:

- Hardening and furring up of the arteries
- Coronary heart disease
- Cataracts
- Premature ageing of the skin
- Chronic inflammatory diseases such as arthritis
- Impaired immunity
- Cancerous changes in cells
- Poor sperm count and poor sperm quality
- Congenital birth defects

Antioxidant vitamins and minerals are the body's main defence against free radical attack. They quickly neutralize the negative charge on a free radical before it can trigger a chain reaction.

Eat more plant-based hormones

One of the most helpful changes you can make is to eat more of the types of plant that contain weak, oestrogen-like chemicals. These mimic the effects of your own oestrogen hormones and can help to reduce symptoms linked with the menopause and possibly premenstrual syndrome. Plants containing oestrogen-like hormones include:

- Legumes, especially soya beans, chickpeas, lentils, alfalfa, mung beans.
- Vegetables: dark-green leafy vegetables (for example, broccoli, pak choi, spinach) and exotic members of the cruciferous family (for example, chinese leaves, kohl rabi); celery, fennel.
- Nuts: almonds, cashew nuts, hazelnuts, peanuts, walnuts and nut oils.
- Seeds, especially linseeds, pumpkin, sesame, sunflower and sprouted seeds.
- Wholegrains: almost all, especially corn, buckwheat, millet, oats, rye, wheat.
- Fresh fruits: apples, avocados, bananas, mangoes, papayas, rhubarb.
- Dried fruits, especially dates, figs, prunes, raisins.
- Culinary herbs: especially angelica, chervil, chives, garlic, ginger, horseradish, nutmeg, parsley, rosemary and sage.

Herbal supplements

Many herbal dietary supplements are helpful during times of stress, especially those that act as adaptogens. An adaptogen is a substance that strengthens, normalizes and regulates all the body's systems. It has wide-ranging beneficial actions and boosts immunity through several different actions to help you adapt to a wide variety of new or stressful situations. Many adaptogens have been shown to normalize blood-sugar levels, hormone imbalances, disrupted biorhythms and the physical and emotional effects of stress.

Ginseng

Ginseng – usually referred to as Chinese, Korean or American ginseng (*Panax ginseng; P. quinquefolius*) – is a perennial plant native to northeast China, North Korea and eastern Russia.

Ginseng has been used in the Orient as a revitalizing adaptogen for over 7,000 years. It is especially helpful during times of stress as it contains plant substances that support the function of the adrenal glands when they are overworked. Clinical trials confirm that ginseng helps the body adapt to physical or emotional stress and fatigue. It is stimulating and restorative, improving physical and mental energy, stamina, strength, alertness and concentration. Those taking ginseng have faster reaction times than when not taking it, and it improves stamina while reducing muscle cramps and fatigue.

Make sure you buy a good quality product from a reputable

company, or one standardized to contain at least 7 per cent ginseno-sides. This will generally be more expensive, but cheap versions may contain very little active ingredient.

Self-help

- The dose depends on the grade of root. Choose a standardized product, preferably with a content of at least 5 per cent ginsenosides for American ginseng and 15 per cent ginsenosides for Korean ginseng. Start with a low dose and work up from 200 to 1000 mg per day until you find a dose that suits you. 1000 mg may be too stimu-lating, so 600 mg is often ideal. The optimum dose is usually around 600 mg daily. Ginseng should not be taken for more than six weeks without a break. In the East, it is taken in a two weeks on, two weeks off cycle. Some practitioners recommend taking it in a six weeks on, eight weeks off cycle.

- Ginseng is not advised if you have high blood pressure (it may make hypertension worse), glaucoma or have an oestrogen-dependent condition (for example, pregnancy, cancer of the breast, ovaries or uterus) as it contains oestrogenic compounds.

- It is best to avoid taking other stimulants such as caffeine-containing products and drinks while taking ginseng. When taken in therapeu-tic doses in a two weeks on, two weeks off cycle, side effects should not be a problem. If you find Chinese ginseng too stimulating, however, you could try American ginseng which seems to have a more gentle action.

- American ginseng is said to be best for fatigue caused by nervous conditions, anxiety and insomnia, while Korean ginseng is better for fatigue with general weakness and loss of energy.

Siberian ginseng

Siberian ginseng *(Eleutherococcus senticosus)* is a deciduous shrub native to eastern Russia, China, Korea and Japan. Its root has similar actions to that of Korean and American *(Panax)* ginsengs, but it is not closely related.

Siberian ginseng is one of the most widely researched herbal adaptogens. It is used extensively to improve stamina and strength, particularly during or after illness and when suffering from other forms of stress and fatigue. Russian research suggests that as a result of boosting immunity, those taking it regularly have 40 per cent less colds, flu and other infections compared with previous winters, and take a third less days off work due to health problems than those not taking it.

Self-help

- Choose a brand that is standardized to contain more than 1 per cent of eleutherosides and take 1000–2000 mg in capsule form per day. Occasionally up to 6000 mg daily is recommended. It is traditionally taken for two to three weeks followed by a two-week break for those who are generally young, healthy and fit. Those who are older, weaker or unwell may take their doses continuously. Take on an empty stomach unless it is too relaxing, in which case take it with meals.

- As with Panax ginseng, Siberian ginseng is best taken cyclically. Take daily for two to three months, then have a month without. Most people begin to notice a difference after around five days, but continue to take it for at least one month for the full restorative effect.

- No serious side effects have been reported. Do not use (except under medical advice) if you suffer from high blood pressure, a tendency to nose bleeds, heavy periods, insomnia, rapid heartbeat (tachycardia), high fever or congestive heart failure. Do not take during pregnancy or when breastfeeding except under specific medical advice.

Ginkgo

The *Ginkgo biloba*, or maidenhair tree, is one of the most popular health supplements in Europe and can improve memory and concentration as well as increasing peripheral blood flow. It is also helpful for stress-induced anxiety, depression and migraine.

Self-help

- Choose extracts standardized for at least 24 per cent ginkolides and take 40–60 mg two or three times a day (take a minimum of 120 mg daily). Stimulating effects last from three to six hours but they may not be noticed until after ten days of treatment.

Gotu kola

Gotu kola *(Centella asiatica)* is a perennial plant native to the Orient. It is known in India as *brahmi* and is one of the most important ayurvedic herbs, used to relieve anxiety and depression, improve memory, promote calm (in larger doses), relax muscle tension, boost adrenal function during times of stress and relieve pain. It is also said to increase physical and mental energy levels.

Self-help

- Choose extracts standardized to contain 25 mg triterpenes, and take two to four capsules daily.
- No serious side effects have been reported. High doses may cause headaches. Large doses are calming rather than energizing.

Garlic

Garlic *(Allium sativum)* is a popular culinary herb that has antibacterial and antiviral actions. Clinical trials using standardized tablets have shown that taking garlic regularly can reduce high blood pressure, lower levels of harmful blood fats (LDL-cholesterol and triglycerides), reduce blood stickiness and improve circulation to all parts of the body. Regular use reduces the risk of hardening and furring up of the arteries up to 25 per cent, and garlic is therefore an important protective herb for those under stress who are at increased risk of high blood pressure and coronary heart disease.

Self-help

- Take 600–900 mg standardized garlic-powder tablets per day.
- Garlic products made by solvent extraction or by boiling garlic in oil are less effective than tablets made from garlic that has been freeze-dried and powdered.

St John's wort

St John's wort *(Hypericum perforatum)* is an effective and gentle anti-depressant that can help to overcome many of the emotional effects of stress. It can lift low moods in at least 67 per cent of those with mild to moderate depression.

Self-help

- Hypericum is best taken with food. Choose extracts standardized to 0.3 per cent hypericin and take 300 mg three times a day.
- Side effects are significantly less likely than with standard antidepressants. Those reported include indigestion, allergic reactions, restlessness and tiredness/fatigue, each in less than 1 per cent of people. Do not take during pregnancy or when breastfeeding. Do not take together with other antidepressants except under medical supervision.
- It is best to avoid alcohol when taking hypericum. Those who are sun-sensitive should also avoid exposing their skin directly to sunlight while taking it – especially if fair-skinned.

4 TAKE EXERCISE AND RELAX

Once you have taken your life and diet in hand, look towards increasing the amount of exercise you take each week. Start with some relaxation exercises, the core of which is breathing technique. Don't forget to include other forms of activity to boost your heart rate.

The power of relaxation

The way you breathe reflects the amount of stress you are under. When you feel relaxed, your breathing will be calm and regular (10–14 breaths per minute) and you will move your whole rib cage and diaphragm. When you feel anxious, however, your breathing rate speeds up to 15–20 breaths per minute and your breaths become shallow (involving the upper part of your rib cage only) and irregular, interspersed with deep sighs and gasps as you try to get more air. The signs of a poor breathing habit are:

- Rapid, shallow breathing involving the upper part of the chest only.
- Shoulders rise significantly towards the ears.

- No visible expansion of the abdomen. Irregular breathing pattern with lots of deep sighs.
- Air-gulping, which leads to abdominal wind and belching.
- Taking deep breaths and holding on to them without breathing out.

Healthy breathing check

To help you recognize what normal, gentle breathing feels like:

1. Lie down and make yourself comfortable and relaxed.
2. Rest your hands on the upper part of your chest.
3. Breathe gently in and out for about a minute and feel the way your chest rises and falls.
4. Now place your hands on your rib cage so your fingertips almost touch when you breathe out.
5. Focusing your attention on when you breathe out rather than when you breathe in, breathe gently for another minute or so and feel your rib cage as it moves upwards and outwards each time.
6. Finally, place your hands on your abdomen with your fingertips just touching. Breathe gently for another minute and feel your fingers part as your abdomen rises and falls.
7. Continue breathing gently and hold on to the calm feeling.

Repeat this breathing exercise daily until you recognize how slow, gentle breathing should feel.

When you are under long-term excess pressure, it is easy for bad breathing habits to build up. By consciously changing the way you breathe, you can help to switch off some of the effects of the stress response and reduce feelings of anxiety.

The following exercise is useful to help you control your breathing when you feel stressed, or to relax before meditation or visualization.

Breathing Exercise 1

1. Sit back comfortably, with your arms hanging loosely at your sides.

2. Breathe in slowly and deeply, concentrating on the rise and fall of your abdomen rather than your chest.

3. When you reach your limit of breathing in, immediately start to breath out to empty your lungs as much as possible.

4. Get your rhythm right by slowly counting up to three when breathing in and slowly counting up to four when breathing out.

5. Repeat the exercise five times without holding your breath.

Breathing Exercise 2

1. Change your breathing rhythm if necessary to ensure that breathing out always takes longer than breathing in.

2. Gradually increase the length of exhalation until inhalation is short (2–3 seconds) and exhalation takes 7–8 seconds in a slow, continuous movement. Place your hands on your chest or abdomen, as described in the 'Healthy breathing check' on page

155, if this helps you to feel your breathing movements.

3. Concentrate on emptying your lungs and on keeping the air movement continuous – don't breathe out all your air quickly and wait for the end of the count to breathe in. It will take practice to slow down to this rate of about six breaths per minute.

Once you have learned this technique and feel able to control your breathing, you will find it invaluable for calming rising panic.

Yoga

Yoga is a gentle and ancient form of oriental exercise that uses posture, breathing techniques and relaxation to increase suppleness and vitality, calm the body, improve sleep and relieve stress. Several different types of yoga exist and hatha yoga, which concentrates on posture and exercise, is the one most widely practised in the West. As with all therapies, it is best to receive training from a qualified teacher, who will help you achieve mental control and the right yoga positions for you. Yoga is based on the concept that physical exercises are linked to mental and spiritual development. Breathing is a major element since the breath embodies a person's *prana* or life-force, and plays an important role in helping problems associated with emotional and mental disharmony. Many yoga exercises and positions will help control the rapid breathing of hyperventilation, while the stretching and relaxing of muscles is a wonderful way to start or end the day, particularly for those experiencing stress, insomnia and anxiety.

Before starting there are a few points to make sure of:

- Check with your doctor if you have a back problem or high blood pressure.
- Do not use yoga within an hour of eating – wait three hours after a heavy meal.
- Empty your bladder and bowel.
- Don't mix yoga with smoking, drugs or alcohol.
- Wear comfortable, light clothing that stretches easily.

T'ai chi ch'uan

T'ai chi ch'uan – often known as t'ai chi – means 'the supreme way of the fist'. It is a Chinese therapy that uses slow, graceful movements, meditation and breathing techniques to achieve total body control, improve the flow of the life-energy force, or *chi*, and to calm the mind. It is sometimes described as meditation in motion. It is a non-combative form of martial arts that stimulates the mind and body.

Research confirms that t'ai chi can reduce stress and that, as a form of exercise, it can improve breathing efficiency. It is important to learn t'ai chi from a teacher if possible, although training videos are available.

Sessions start with a gentle warm-up exercise and are ideally performed every day.

Exercise and weight

Before moving onto developing an exercise regime (see page 163) assess your weight and overall shape because this will help determine how much exercise you should take and at what level you should start.

Are you an apple or a pear?

Work out your waist:hip ratio by measuring your waist and hips in centimetres, then divide the waist measurement by the hip measurement to produce your ratio. For example, if your waist measures 99 cm and your hips 109 cm, your waist:hip ratio is 99 divided by 109, which is 0.9.

- If you are female, is your waist:hip ratio less than 0.85?
- If you are male, is your waist:hip ratio less than 0.95?

If it is, you're 'pear-shaped'; if not, you're 'apple-shaped'.

People who are apple-shaped have a higher risk of hardening and furring up of the arteries, high cholesterol levels, high blood pressure, coronary heart disease, stroke and diabetes than those who are pear-shaped. The reason is not fully understood, but is probably linked with the way your body handles dietary fats. Lack of exercise and drinking excessive amounts of alcohol also seem to encourage fat gain around the waist. People who are under stress and also apple-shaped therefore need to take urgent steps to increase their level of activity. Luckily, people who are apple-shaped seem to lose weight more easily than those who are pear-shaped. This is because abdominal fat is mobilized and broken down more easily than fat stored elsewhere.

If you are overweight and also apple-shaped, you have a high risk of developing coronary heart disease – especially if this runs in your family. In fact, waist size alone may be a good indicator of health – or lack of it. New research suggests that men with a waist circumference larger than 102 cm and women with a waist circumference larger than 88 cm are more likely to have shortness of breath, high blood pressure, high cholesterol levels and diabetes than those with slimmer waistlines. Slight waist reductions of just 5–10 cm significantly reduced the risk of having a heart attack.

Are you in the healthy weight range?

Using a calculator, work out your body mass index (BMI) – this is assessed by dividing your weight in kilograms by the square of your height in metres. For example, someone with a weight of 70 kg and a height of 1.7 m has a BMI of $70 \div 1.7 \div 1.7 = 24.22$ kg/m^2.

The calculation produces a number that can be interpreted by the table below.

BMI	Weight band
< 20	underweight
20-25	healthy
25-30	overweight
30-40	obese
> 40	morbidly obese

OPTIMUM HEALTHY WEIGHT RANGE

HEIGHT Metres/feet	MEN Kg	Stones	WOMEN Kg	Stones
1.47/4'10"			40–51	6st 4–8st
1.50/4'11"			42–54	6st 8–8st 7
1.52/5ft			43–55	6st 11–8st 9
1.55/5'1"			45–57	7st 1–8st 13
1.57/5'2"			46–59	7st 3–9st 4
1.60/5'3"			48–61	7st 8–9st 8
1.63/5'4"			50–63	7st 12–9st 13
1.65/5'5"			51–65	8st–10st 3
1.68/5'6"	56–70	8st 12–11 st	53–67	8st 5–10st 7
1.70/5'7"	58–72	9st 1–11st 4	54–69	8st 7–10st 12
1.73/5'8"	60–75	9st 6–11st 10	56–71	8st 11–11st 2
1.75/5'9"	61–76	9st 9 –12st	57–73	8st 13–11st 7
1.78/5'10"	63–79	9st 1–12st 6	59–75	9st 4–11st 11
1.80/5'11"	65–81	10st 3–12st 9	61–77	9st 8–12st 1
1.83/6ft	67–83	10st 7–13st 1	63–80	9st 13–12st 8
1.85/6'1"	69–85	10st 11–13st 5		
1.88/6'2"	71–88	11st 2–13st 12		
1.90/6'3"	72–90	11st 5–14st 2		
1.93/6'4"	75–93	11st 10–14st 8		

If your BMI is in the overweight range (25–30), you should try to lose a few pounds to bring you back into the healthy weight range for your height. Those who are overweight are one-and-a-half times more likely to have a heart attack than someone who maintains a healthy weight. Where excess weight is stored is also important. If you are overweight and also store fat round your middle (apple-shaped), you are twice as likely to develop coronary heart disease – especially if this runs in your family. Getting down to the healthy weight range for your height can reduce your risk of a heart attack by as much as 35–55 per cent.

The chart on the previous page shows the optimum healthy weight range that you should aim for, for your height. The figures for women are slightly stricter than for men (a BMI of 18.7–23.8 for women, and 20–25 for men) to take account of their different muscle:fat ratio.

As well as helping to reduce an apple shape and helping you lose weight, exercise increases your strength (by building up muscle bulk), your stamina (by increasing muscle energy stores), and your suppleness (by improving the range of movement of joints and making ligaments and tendons more flexible). Increased stamina is particularly important when you are under stress.

Exercise and stress

Exercise burns off the effects of adrenaline and helps to neutralize the fight-or-flight response and return your systems to their rest/digest setting. Regular exercise can boost your immunity and even prolong your life. A study of more than 10,000 men found that exercise reduced the number of age-related deaths from all causes by almost a quarter – even if exercise was not started until middle age. Regular exercise is therefore essential for those experiencing high levels of stress.

Unfortunately, seven out of ten men and eight out of ten women do not take enough exercise to have a beneficial effect on their heart or to reduce their levels of stress. Ideally, you should exercise briskly for 20 or 30 minutes five times a week. Once you are fit, exercise every day.

Starting an exercise regime

If you are relatively unfit, don't launch straight into a jogging programme. To achieve fitness, start off slowly and take regular exercise lasting for 20 or 30 minutes, for a minimum of five times per week (for example, two days' exercise, one day's rest). Once you have achieved a reasonable level of fitness, you should do more.

Your level of exercise should be strenuous enough to work up a slight sweat and to make you slightly breathless. Always warm up first with a few simple bends and stretches, and cool down afterwards by walking slowly for a few minutes. If you have problems with your joints (for example, arthritis) or find it difficult to manage a brisk walk, try a non-weight-bearing form of exercise such as cycling or swimming.

The golden rule is, if it hurts – stop. If at any time you become so breathless that you can't speak, develop chest tightness or pain, or feel dizzy or unwell, stop immediately and seek medical advice. If you have a heart problem, you should seek medical advice before embarking on a physical exercise programme.

Self-help

- Take up an active hobby such as ballroom dancing, bowls, swimming, golf, walking or cycling.

- If you dislike exercise, try to put more effort into DIY or gardening.

- Spend less time watching TV and more time pottering in the garden or around the house – listen to music or the radio if you like background noise.

- Walk up stairs rather than using the lift or escalator.

- Walk or cycle reasonable distances rather than taking the car.

- Walk around the block in your lunch hour.

- If you can't go out, try walking up and down stairs a few times a day.

- Reintroduce the traditional habit of a family walk after Sunday lunch.

- Start getting up an hour earlier than usual and go for a walk, cycle, do some gardening, fetch the daily paper or visit the gym.

- Buy a home exercise machine and use it while watching the evening news.

Swimming

Swimming is an excellent cardiovascular exercise as it involves just about every muscle in your body and rapidly builds stamina, strength and suppleness. To get the most benefit from swimming, try to develop a variety of different strokes and indulge at least two or three times a week, and preferably every day. Swimming is a non-weight-bearing form of exercise that is excellent for those with joint problems. The fact that you are exercising against the weight of water means it is also good for building up muscle strength.

Aqua aerobics

Aqua aerobics is a fun form of exercise that makes use of the 'weight' of water to exercise your muscles more than on dry land. It is excellent for those who do not enjoy swimming lengths. Most swimming pools hold regular classes.

Walking

Brisk walking is an excellent form of exercise, especially when carried out in bracing country air. Walking boosts your stamina and can help to burn off the effects of stress. A beginner should aim to walk a mile in around 20 minutes, increasing to three miles in about 50 minutes after about three months. Walking briskly (4.5 miles per hour) for 30 minutes burns up 200 calories – enough to lose 1 lb every two weeks if you do it each day.

Invest in a good pair of walking shoes with cushioned soles and some ankle support to protect your feet and lower joints. Always warm up first with a few simple bends and stretches. Cool down afterwards by walking slowly for a few minutes.

To maintain your new fitness level, try to take at least 30 minutes' exercise three times a week.

Cycling

Cycling is efficient at improving strength, stamina and suppleness. It is a low-impact, non-weight-bearing aerobic activity which, like swimming, doesn't put your muscles, ligaments or joints under excessive strain. This makes cycling particularly good for the overweight or those with joint problems. Cycling can be performed at home with a machine, in the gym or outdoors. Studies have shown that people who exercise in the fresh air derive greater benefits and get fitter quicker. Start off with a low gear ratio to keep resistance low and concentrate on pedalling technique and speed. As your stamina increases, introduce more intense bursts of exercise to increase your fitness.

SUGGESTED CYCLING REGIMES

In the gym

The average non-fit person should start off on an exercise bike using a simple regime. A trainer will help you to tailor a cycling regime to suit your fitness goals.

Out and about

If you own your own bike, it is important to be aware of cycling safety:

- use lights at dusk
- fit a red reflector to the rear mudguard and amber reflectors to your pedals
- maintain and oil your bike regularly
- wear reflective clothing at night
- avoid roads where there is fast or heavy traffic
- consider taking a cycling proficiency test
- always wear a safety helmet that complies with current safety standards

Initially, cycle during the day on a route you know well where there are plenty of other people about and little traffic. Keep to level ground for the first few weeks, then slowly introduce gentle hills. When you feel up to it, try cycling up steeper inclines.

To maintain your new fitness level, continue cycling three or four times per week. Try to average at least three hours of brisk exercise spread out over each seven-day period.

5 EXPLORE ALTERNATIVE THERAPIES

Alternative therapies are becoming increasingly popular and accepted as a viable alternative to conventional medicine. They use an holistic approach that treats the mind, body and spirit rather than isolated symptoms, and this can be especially helpful in overcoming stress. More and more people now realize that a healthy body stems from healthy emotions, and by encouraging a more positive frame of mind, complementary techniques offer a gentler form of healing.

The following alternative therapies have helped many people with stress, but just as with orthodox medicine, not every treatment will suit every individual. This chapter gives an overview of the most popular alternative therapies. For more detailed advice seek out a specialist practioner (see Resources, page 218).

Choosing an alternative practitioner

Bear in mind that standards of training and experience vary widely. Where possible:

- Select a therapist on the basis of personal recommendation from a satisfied client whom you know and whose opinion you trust.

- Check what qualifications the therapist has, and check their standing with the relevant umbrella organization for that therapy. The organization will be able to tell you what training their members have undertaken, what their code of ethics is, and refer you to qualified practitioners in your area.

- Find out how long your course of treatment will last and how much it is likely to cost.

- Ask how much experience the practitioner has had in treating stress and what their success rate is.

Acupuncture

Acupuncture is based on the belief that life energy (*qi* or *chi* – pronounced 'chee') flows through the body along different channels known as meridians. This flow of energy depends on the balance of two opposing forces: yin and yang – a balance that is easily disrupted through factors such as stress, anger, poor diet, spiritual neglect and even the weather. There are 12 main meridians – six of which have a yang polarity and are related to hollow organs (for example, the stomach), and six are yin and relate mainly to solid organs (for example, the liver). These 12 meridians are controlled by a further two: the 'conception' and 'governing' vessels.

Each meridian has a number of acupuncture points (acupoints) overlying it where chi energy is concentrated and can enter or leave the body. Traditionally, 365 acupoints were described, but more have been discovered in modern times and now around 2000 acupoints are illustrated on charts. When the flow of chi energy becomes blocked or imbalanced, symptoms of illness or emotional disturbances are triggered. By inserting fine needles into acupuncture points overlying these meridians, the flow of chi energy can be stimulated or suppressed to overcome blockages or imbalances associated with various symptoms. A therapist will select which acupoints to access depending on your individual symptoms, the appearance of your tongue, and on the quality, rhythm and strength of 12 pulses (six in each wrist). These represent the 12 main organs and functions in acupuncture, and help to identify areas where the flow of chi is blocked.

Fine, disposable stainless-steel needles are inserted which cause little, if any, discomfort. You may notice a slight pricking sensation, or an odd tingling buzz as the needle is inserted a few millimetres into the skin. The needles are usually left in place from a few minutes to half an hour, and may be periodically flicked to enhance the quality of *chi*, or vigorously rotated to stir up a stagnant *chi* and draw or disperse energy from the point. Sometimes, a small cone of dried herb (moxa – usually mugwort, *Artemesia vulgaris*) is ignited and burned near the active acupoint (or attached to a copper-handled needle) to warm the skin. This is known as moxibustion. It is believed that the warmth stimulates energy in areas that are cold or painful because *chi* is weak.

Most patients start to notice a benefit after four to six treatments. Sometimes you may feel worse at first, which suggests your energies have been over-stimulated. Let the therapist know, as they will need to use fewer needles for a shorter length of time during your next treatment.

Acupressure

Acupressure is an ancient skill that has been practised in China and Japan for over 3000 years. It is similar to acupuncture, but instead of inserting needles at points along the meridians, these are stimulated using firm thumb pressure or fingertip massage. Sometimes the therapist will use their palms, elbows, knees and feet to massage and balance the flow of *chi* energy throughout your body. The best known example of acupressure is Japanese shiatsu – meaning 'finger pressure'.

You can use acupressure on yourself to help relieve minor stress-related conditions but more specialist treatments should be performed by a trained therapist. Only a specialist should use acupressure on someone who is pregnant.

When energy flow becomes abnormal, acupoints on the surrounding skin become tender and painful to touch. These are known as tsubos and are important areas to which acupressure or acupuncture treatments can be applied.

Aromatherapy

Aromatherapy harnesses the beneficial properties of aromatic essential oils produced by special glands in the leaves, flowers, fruit and seeds of medicinal plants. These essential oils can help to treat a variety of conditions but are particularly effective for stress or emotional problems since they can produce a powerful effect on your moods. Aromatherapy oils directly stimulate the sense of smell, which is connected with a part of the brain (the limbic system) closely involved in regulating the emotions. Oils are also absorbed from the skin into the circulation and can have powerful effects on the body. Too much of them can be harmful and it is important that oils are chosen with care and used according to the instructions.

Where possible, use natural rather than synthetic essential oils: they have a fuller, sweeter aroma that is of greater therapeutic benefit. Similarly, 100 per cent pure essential oils are preferable – although they are usually more expensive – since they are not mixed with alcohol or other additives.

Using essential oils

- Aromatherapy essential oils may be inhaled, massaged into the skin, added to bath water, or heated in a variety of ways to perfume the atmosphere.

- Oils that come into contact with skin should always be diluted with

Cautions

- Do not take essential oils internally.
- Before using an essential oil blend on your skin, do a patch test (put a small amount on a patch of skin and leave it for at least an hour) to make sure you are not sensitive to it.
- Do not use essential oils if you are pregnant, or likely to be, except under specialist advice from a qualified aromatherapist.
- Do not use essential oils if you suffer from epilepsy, except under specialist advice from a qualified aromatherapist.
- Avoid using aromatherapy oils that are known to be capable of putting blood pressure up. These include thyme, clove and cinnamon.
- Keep essential oils away from the eyes.
- If you are taking homeopathic remedies, do not use peppermint, rosemary or lavender essential oils as these may neutralize the homeopathic effect.
- Essential oils are flammable, so do not put them near an open flame.

a carrier oil (for example, almond, avocado, jojoba or wheatgerm oil). Dilution is important as oils that are too concentrated may have an adverse effect or cause skin irritation. Add a maximum total of one drop of essential oil to each 2 ml (24 drops) of carrier oil. Two teaspoons (10 ml) of carrier oil should therefore contain no more than 5 drops of essential oil blend, while 2 tablespoons (30 ml) should contain no more than 15 drops of essential oil blend.

- Oils that are twice as dilute as this often suffice (i.e., only 5 drops of essential oil blend per 20 ml of carrier oil). A 5 ml medicinal teaspoon measure (or a 5 ml syringe if you prefer) can be bought cheaply from a chemist to ensure accuracy; kitchen teaspoons tend to hold slightly less than 5 ml.

- To make a relaxing massage oil add a maximum total of one drop of essential oil to each 2 ml (24 drops) of carrier oil.

- To add to your bath: Add 5 drops of essential oils to a tablespoon of carrier oil and mix. Draw your bath so that it is comfortably hot, then add the aromatic oil mix after the taps are turned off. Close the bathroom door to keep in the vapours and soak yourself for 15–20 minutes, preferably by candlelight.

- In the shower: Add 8 drops of essential oil to a tablespoon (15 ml) of carrier oil. After cleansing your body with soap or gel, rinse well then dip a wet sponge in the oil mix and use it to gently massage your whole body while under a warm jet spray.

- To help you sleep: Add 2 or 3 drops of a relaxing oil blend to a tissue and allow to dry before tucking under your pillow.

- With a candlelit diffuser: Add 2 or 3 drops of essential oil to a little warm water over a candle burner to diffuse oils into a room.

- With an electric ionizer/diffuser: Buy an ionizer/diffuser that has a hot plate on to which you add oils or oils mixed with water.

Ayurveda

Indian medicine, known as ayurveda or 'the science of life', is one of the oldest forms of holistic medicine, and can be dated back to almost 5000 years ago. The body, like the universe, is said to be made up of five elements: earth, ether (space), fire, water and air, which make up three internal forces or *doshas*, known as *pitta*, *kapha* and *vata* (the driving force, seated in the colon). Each person has one (and occasionally two) dominant *doshas*, which determine their constitution and the type of illnesses to which they are susceptible. The level of each *dosha* is said to rise and fall according to the time of day, the season, the type of diet you eat, the stresses you are under, and the extent of repressed emotions. When the *doshas* become unbalanced, they are thought to block the flow of the life-force *prana*, which is comparable with the Chinese life-force, *chi*. During times of stress, the three *doshas* become unbalanced, leading to disease.

Ayurveda may use a variety of techniques to help relieve stress and bring internal balance in the doshas. These include diet, meditation, posture control, breathing exercises, yoga, hydrotherapy and herbal medicines. One of ayurveda's main doctrines is that prevention is better than cure, so changes will be suggested in your diet and lifestyle to help stop levels of stress from rising.

By balancing your internal systems, ayurveda can help you achieve emotional and physical health and can treat the symptoms of stress, as well as maintaining good health in those who are unstressed.

Bach Flower Remedies

Flower Remedies were devised earlier this century when Dr Edward
Bach noticed that patients suffering from the same emotional problems
benefited from the same homeopathic treatment, irrespective of the
physical symptoms they were suffering. He came to believe that physical
disease was due to underlying emotional stresses that would inevitably
lead to more serious illness in the future. Using his medical skills, he
classified emotional problems into seven major groups, which were
further subdivided into a total of 38 negative or harmful states of mind.
Using his homeopathic skills, he then formulated a series of plant-based
remedies to treat these emotional conditions, correcting the harmful
states of mind and restoring emotional balance before the adverse
effects of stress led to physical disease.

Bach Flower Remedies are prepared either by infusion or boiling. In
the infusion method, flower heads are placed on the surface of a small
glass bowl filled with pure spring water. This is left to infuse in direct
sunlight for three hours, then the flowers are discarded and the infused
spring water is preserved in grape alcohol (brandy). This resultant
solution is called the mother tincture and is further diluted five times to
create the individual stock remedies.

In the boiling method, short lengths of twig bearing flowers or
catkins are boiled in pure spring water for 30 minutes. The plant
material is then discarded and the water allowed to cool before being
preserved in grape alcohol to produce a mother tincture.

Using a Flower Remedy

- Add two drops of it to any-sized glass of mineral or spring water, or fruit juice. Sip and hold each mouthful in the mouth for a few seconds before swallowing.

- For emergency situations (for example, panic attacks, just before public speaking) use Rescue Remedy, which is a composite of five remedies: rock rose, impatiens, clematis, star-of-Bethlehem and cherry plum. Add four drops to a glass of liquid and sip slowly every few minutes until symptoms subside. Hold each sip in your mouth for a moment before swallowing.

- If no fluid is available, remedies may also be dropped directly on to the tongue or rubbed on to the lips, behind the ears or elsewhere on the body.

Craniosacral therapy

Craniosacral therapy is a modern version of cranial osteopathy that involves the gentle laying on of hands, mainly over the skull and lower spine. Experienced therapists assess the flow of cerebrospinal fluid (known as the cranial rhythmic impulse) and 'listen' to the inner movements and tensions within the patient. Due to the continuity of fluids and tissues in the body, the laying on of hands releases inner energy and tensions to produce relaxation and healing. Craniosacral therapy is able to help headaches, migraines, TMJ (temporomandibular joint) syndrome and other stress-related aches and pains using a holistic rather than a symptom-orientated approach. Most people experiencing craniosacral therapy feel deeply relaxed during the treatment and experience a spontaneous unwinding of tension due to the release of physical and emotional imbalances. It is not a technique you can perform on yourself.

Homeopathy

Homeopathy is based on the belief that natural substances can boost the body's own healing powers to relieve symptoms and signs of illness. Substances are selected which, if used full-strength, would produce symptoms in a healthy person similar to those it is designed to treat. This is the first principle of homeopathy, that 'like cures like'. The second major principle of homeopathy is that increasing the dilution of a solution has the opposite effect of increasing its potency: 'less cures more'. By diluting noxious and even poisonous substances many millions of times, their healing properties are enhanced while their undesirable side effects are lost.

On the centesimal scale, dilutions of 100^{-6} are described as potencies of 6c, dilutions of 100^{-30} are written as a potency of 30c, and so on. At these levels of dilution, the homeopathic remedies are no longer dilutions but biophysically altered solutions. A dilution of 12c (100^{-12}) is comparable to a pinch of salt dissolved in the same amount of water as is found in the Atlantic Ocean.

Homeopathy is thought to work in a dynamic way, boosting your body's own healing powers. The most popular theory to explain how homeopathy works is that the original noxious substance added to the water somehow left a footprint in the solution that the body can recognize and respond to. Over 2000 homeopathic remedies are available. It is best to see a trained homeopath who can assess your con-stitutional type, personality, lifestyle, family background, likes and dislikes as well as your symptoms before deciding which treatment is right for you. Some homeopathic treatments are selected according to emotional traits such as anger, timidity, anxiety or depression, important in treating stress-related problems.

Homeopathic remedies may be prescribed by a medically-trained homeopathic doctor on the normal NHS prescription form and dispensed by homeopathic pharmacists for the usual prescription charge or exemptions. Alternatively, you can consult a private homeopathic practitioner or buy remedies direct from a pharmacist.

Using homeopathic remedies

- Homeopathic remedies should ideally be taken on their own, without eating or drinking for at least thirty minutes before or after.

- Tablets should also be taken without handling – tip them into the lid of the container, or on to a teaspoon to transfer them into your mouth. Then suck or chew them, don't swallow them whole.

- If there is no obvious improvement after taking the remedies for the time stated, consult a practitioner. Don't be surprised if your symptoms initially get worse before they get better – persevere through this common reaction to treatment; it is a good sign which shows the remedy is working.

- After completing a course of homeopathy, you will usually feel much better, with a greatly improved sense of well-being that lets you cope with any remaining symptoms in a much more positive way.

Hydrotherapy

Hydrotherapy – or the use of water in healing – is a popular technique that takes a wide variety of forms. Bathing in essential oils, mineral solutions, seaweed extracts, mud, peat, hot spas and sea water have been used for medicinal purposes since ancient times.

Temperature plays an important role, with cold baths used to stimulate metabolism and boost immunity, warm water used for floatation therapy, and hot water to treat muscle aches and joint pains as well as generally to soothe, relax and heal. The ancient Greeks believed in the use of a sitz bath in which the bottom was immersed in a hip bath of one temperature, and the feet in a bowl of water at a different temperature.

Thalassotherapy is a form of hydrotherapy based on the healing properties of sea water and seaweed. Seaweed extracts are added to baths or used as body wraps and poultices to encourage sweating and to draw impurities out of the skin. Seaweed is rich in trace elements and minerals, some of which can be absorbed by the skin – people who are allergic to iodine should therefore avoid this therapy.

While everyone uses the bath and shower at home for cleansing, a daily immersion ritual also has a therapeutic effect and – especially if combined with candlelight and aromatherapy oils at the end of a stressful day – can be immensely relaxing.

Self-help

- When using any of the following treatments, don't get up too quickly from the bath as your blood pressure may temporarily drop low enough to make you feel faint. Do not use the following treatments if you are pregnant, within two hours of a heavy meal or if you have been drinking alcohol.

- Add a sachet (around 450 g) of Dead Sea salts to a warm bath and relax for twenty minutes. Then wrap yourself in a warm towel and lie on a bed in a warm room for a deeply relaxing experience. (NB Do not allow the salts to get in your eyes. Cover cuts or grazes with Vaseline or they will sting.)

- Add 450 g Epsom salts to a warm-to-medium hot bath and relax for ten minutes then rinse or wash off the salt water. (NB Do not allow the salts to get in your eyes. Cover cuts or grazes with Vaseline or they will sting.)

- Add diluted camomile, lavender, jasmine, sandalwood or ylang-ylang oils to a bath of warm water and relax for fifteen minutes to help reduce anxiety.

- Add diluted basil, bergamot, camomile, lavender, jasmine, rose, sandalwood or ylang-ylang oils to a bath of warm water and relax for fifteen minutes to help reduce low moods.

- Add diluted camomile, lavender or rose oils to a bath of warm water and relax for fifteen minutes to help overcome insomnia.

- Add camomile, lavender or ylang-ylang to help defuse anger.

Hypnotherapy

Hypnotherapy is a technique in which suggestion is used to help someone in a profoundly relaxed or trance-like state to heal themselves. Hypnotherapy helps to strengthen your resolve and is most commonly used to help people overcome addictive or obsessive behaviour patterns and phobias. Hypnotherapy can also be used to help you gain control over your life by achieving relaxation in times of anxiety and stress.

Self-help

To help you achieve a relaxed state for self-hypnosis, you should first: Use meditation (see page 188) and then breathing exercises (see page 156). Sit quietly and imagine your hands and arms becoming heavier and heavier until you are unable to lift them. Then you can move on to the following steps:

1. Relax in a warm, quiet, dimly lit room where you will not be disturbed. Sit or lie comfortably with your hands and feet apart.

2. Roll your eyes up until you feel them straining and fix your eyes on an imagined (or real) spot on the ceiling.

3. While still fixating on the ceiling, breathe in deeply as far as you can. Hold the breath to a slow count of ten, then exhale as fully as possible while saying quietly to yourself, 'Relax!'. Repeat twice more, holding your breath for as long as possible after breathing in.

4. Breathe in once more then, as you breathe out and tell yourself to relax, let your eyes close.

5. Imagine your body has become weightless and is slowly floating upwards as you feel more and more relaxed.

6. Imagine you have floated to the top of a hill that has ten terraces leading down on to a plain.

7. Let yourself float down to the first terrace while counting backwards from the number five. Again, use your imagination so you really feel yourself there.

8. Keep floating down until you reach the plain at the bottom. Once there, focus on the change you want to make in yourself, for example, 'I am calm and relaxed', 'I am no longer smoking', 'I am coping well' or 'I am self-confident'. Always use the present tense as this is what your subconscious mind responds to best.

9. Use your imagination to feel yourself in your new, stronger role, repeating the positive phrase over and over again.

10. After 10–20 minutes of visualizing the new empowered you, tell yourself that on the count of five you will slowly float back up the hill, open your eyes and feel refreshed. 'One...two...three... four...five...'

Try to practise this self-hypnosis every day. You will soon be able to achieve a state of relaxation wherever and whenever you want, to find your secret inner place of calm and strength to help you overcome stressful situations.

Massage

Massage is one of the oldest alternative therapies and is based on the healing power of touch. It is especially helpful for easing muscle tension, anxiety, high blood pressure, insomnia, low moods and other stress-related symptoms.

There are several different types of massage, which use a variety of touches – stroking, rubbing, pummelling, kneading, wringing and pressure. All are very relaxing and produce physical effects in the blood and lymphatic circulation at the site of treatment. Many people have found that the psychological, emotional, physical and behavioural symptoms of stress can be largely neutralized simply by receiving a weekly therapeutic massage. Massage forms the basis of many other therapies including acupressure, aromatherapy and shiatsu.

How to give an aromatherapy massage

Giving and receiving an aromatherapy massage is a relaxing, pleasurable experience. Massage your partner for 30 minutes, then relax while the touch experience is returned. Choose appropriate stress-relieving oils such as basil, bergamot, camomile, cedarwood, jasmine, lavender, marjoram, orange, rose and ylang-ylang. Do not massage someone within two hours of a heavy meal. Only a qualified masseuse should work on a woman who is pregnant.

1. Choose a firm surface: try lying on several towels spread on the floor (beds, with the exception of a futon, are usually too soft).

2. Remove jewellery and check your fingernails are short enough.

3. Make sure the room is warm and quiet. Soft candlelight and slow, relaxing background music will help to set the right ambience.

4. Ask your partner to lie on their front, and cover them with a large bath towel. Make sure they are comfortable.

5. Warm the massage oil or lotion by rubbing some oil in your hands to warm it before using. If adding extra oil during the massage, warm it before it comes into contact with your partner's skin.

6. Begin with long, flowing, simple strokes that follow the body contours. As a general rule, stroke towards the heart from whichever part of the body you are working on. These areas are most prone to tension: shoulders, arms, neck, and forehead.

7. When you feel confident, start to vary the pressure and length of stroke you use, keeping movements flowing and rhythmic, with one hand in contact with their body at all times. Avoid heavy pressure directly over the spine.

8. Communicate with each other – say what feels good and whether the pressure and timing are right.

9. When you have finished massaging the back, ask your partner to turn over so you can work on their front. Stroke towards the heart and finish by holding your partner's feet for a few seconds since this helps to 'ground' them.

Meditation

Meditation is a discipline in which the power of concentration is used to control thoughts, calm the body and achieve a state of heightened mental or spiritual awareness. By focusing your mind on a particular object or vision, you can screen out distractions and induce a state of profound relaxation and serenity which can reverse the fight-or-flight response and trigger the rest/digest state of calm. Those experienced in meditation can enter a trance-like state in which the brain generates theta waves, which are associated with creativity, visions and profound relaxation. At the same time, muscle tension is reduced and some adepts can also lower their pulse and blood pressure at will. Meditation is an excellent way to help you sleep at the end of a stressful day.

There are several types of meditation, each of which favours different techniques such as concentrating on your breathing rhythm, a universal sound (for example, om), a word or phrase with personal meaning (a mantra), or a physical object (for example, a flickering candle or a vase of fresh flowers) or an image such as a picture of a loved one. Some techniques, such as t'ai chi ch'uan, involve repetitive movements or feeling objects such as pebbles or worry beads – as each object is moved it is felt and counted in a rhythmic and repetitive manner. The distracting object or thought is not important: it's purpose is to help you shut out other intrusions rather than to form the focus of intensive study. Joss sticks are frequently used to help create a relaxed atmosphere.

Posture

It is important to adopt a comfortable, neutral posture when meditating since tension in your muscles or joints will send distracting, stressful messages to your brain and interfere with meditation. Traditional meditative poses include the lotus position from yoga, kneeling as in prayer, sitting erect or standing – they all have one thing in common: they keep your spine straight. Maintaining total immobility helps to enhance self-control and discipline.

Before starting to meditate it helps to have learned how to relax by more orthodox methods such as breathing exercises (see page 156) so you can more easily achieve a tranquil state.

The value of meditation increases the more you practise. Make it a daily activity, for example while lying in bed before drifting off to sleep. You can even integrate meditation into everyday actions by focusing your senses when carrying out simple tasks such as washing your hands.

Meditation through concentration

Sit comfortably in a neutral position with your eyes closed. Breathe slowly and rhythmically while concentrating your mind on an imagined object. If you wish, you can also repeat a silent sound in your mind such as a low-pitched hum. Passively concentrate on the image and sound, pushing away intrusive thoughts so your mind stays focused on the image or sound you have created. At first you will find that external thoughts keep creeping in every few seconds as your mind wanders. Simply acknowledge that this has happened and return to your focus of meditation. With time you will learn to concentrate on your central focus for 10 to 20 minutes. Try to keep as still as possible and resist the urge to move or scratch. This technique is especially helpful when you are feeling stressed and need to switch off – just a few moments spent in your quiet inner realm can reset your stress button and help you relax when all around is in chaos. When you come to the end of your meditation period, take a minute to 'come to' before slowly opening your eyes and greeting the outer world. Stretch and stand up slowly while enjoying your sense of inner peace and relaxation.

Try imagining one of the following objects when meditating to free stress – choose whichever appeals to you most:

- A slowly rotating green sphere
- A glistening, dew-coated yellow flower slowly moving in the breeze
- Bubbles rising in water
- Rivers of colour bathing you in light – start with red, orange and yellow then imagine the cooler colours of the spectrum – green, blue, indigo and violet
- A white cloud floating in an azure-blue sky

Reflexology

Reflexology is a relaxing therapy that relies on the healing power of touch to balance the body's energy. It is based on the principle that points (reflexes) in the hands or, more commonly, the feet are indirectly related to distant parts of the body. The technique originated in ancient China over 5000 years ago and involves stimulating the reflexes through massage and tiny pressure movements to relieve fatigue and stress-related symptoms such as tension, migraine, breathing disorders, premenstrual syndrome and digestive problems. The presence of tenderness and subtle textural changes in the feet can also help the practitioner to diagnose more distant problems.

At the end of each session you will usually feel warm, contented, relaxed and much less stressed. You can buy a variety of mats, rollers, shoes and brushes that stimulate the reflexes for self-help, but if you are unable to visit a therapist, you and a friend or partner can easily learn to give each other a relaxing foot massage. Use a little aromatherapy oil to make the experience more therapeutic.

How to give a foot massage

1. Hold your partner's foot in both hands for a few moments to allow your auras to interact. Then start stroking the top and bottom of the foot by moving both hands from the toes towards the ankles and back again. Use a light, firm motion and repeat several times to warm the skin.

2. Holding the foot firmly, gently rotate and rock it from side to side and round and round to explore the range of movement at the ankle.

3. Holding the foot still, use your thumbs to apply gentle but firm pressure over the sole of the foot. Cover the whole sole with small circular movements of your thumbs.

4. Repeat the circular thumb massage on the top of the foot and the base of the toes.

5. Holding the foot under the heel with one hand, use the other to gently grasp all the toes and flex the end of the foot up and down.

6. Gently squeeze and massage each toe one at a time, starting with the big toe.

7. Finish by stroking the foot a few times as before, finally letting your fingers slide towards the ends of the toes. Hold the toes for a few moments then gently place the foot on the ground and cover with a towel while you massage the other foot.

Visualization therapy

Visualization is a technique that harnesses the power of the imagination and helps you learn how to boost self-confidence and ease the symptoms of stress. It relies on the power of suggestion and positive thought to visualize a desired outcome. This imagined role-acting then makes it easier to achieve the desired outcome in real life through improved self-awareness and self-confidence. It literally helps you to picture your way out of a stressful situation to achieve relaxation, calm and an elevated mood.

Visualization is similar to meditation but is less structured and easier to perform. It involves entering a relaxed state and allowing your own inner thoughts (or someone else's voice) to guide you on a self-improvement quest or to take you to a quiet place of peace and pleasure. By creating a feeling of contentment and pleasure, the stress fight-or-flight response is switched off and the rest/digest response activated.

Self-help

- Guided visualization most commonly involves the use of a relaxation tape in which you are instructed on how to relax before imagining yourself somewhere pleasant such as in a leafy glade, by a bubbling brook or lying on a sun-drenched tropical beach.

- Unguided visualization uses the same elements as the exercise above, except the journey is replaced by your own wandering thoughts. Imagine looking through a window, for example, and describe what you can see. Then allow your imagination to take you closer so you can see, hear, feel, touch and smell what is happening there. Explore the shapes, sizes, colours and positions of different objects to heighten your senses. Stay in this state for about ten minutes and then bring yourself slowly back to everyday feelings.

- If a particular stress-related symptom is troublesome, picture an image in your mind that represents that symptom, and imagine it away. For example, if you are troubled by tension headaches, visualize the headache as an iron band around your head which gets progressively looser and looser until it falls away.

- One of the most successful visualization techniques is performed just before you go to sleep. This allows your subconscious mind to dwell on what it has learned and improves the chance of a successful outcome. This exercise should involve a visualization that is pertinent to your life, for example if you have an upcoming interview, visualize that going well.

  1. Choose an appropriate positive affirmation, such as 'I am an interesting and confident candidate for the job'.

  2. Every night when you go to bed, imagine yourself greeting the interview panel calmly, dealing logically and confidently with their questions and impressing the board with your knowledge, experience and capabilities.

  3. Feel the confidence growing inside you as you answer all their

questions and make insightful comments on the qualities and benefits you can add to the team.

4. Repeat your positive thought slowly and carefully to yourself.

5. Now touch the bed with the little finger of your left hand. Repeat the thought and touch the bed with the ring finger of your left hand while concentrating on the warm, self-confident feeling of having achieved an excellent interview.

6. Keep repeating Step 5, using each finger (and thumb) of your left hand, and then your right. Then reverse the process, touching the bed starting with the little finger of the right hand. By the time you have finished, you will have repeated the thought twenty times.

Repeat this procedure every night for a week, staying awake throughout the entire process. The following week, repeat the process but let yourself fall asleep when you are ready. The statement should now have become part of your normal thinking patterns.

6 DEVELOP SELF-ESTEEM

To help you take control of your life and develop healthy self-esteem, it helps to learn how to assert yourself, how to think rationally and how to communicate better; and to develop a variety of hobbies and interests outside your work and home life.

Assertiveness

Assertiveness training is based on the underlying belief that everyone is equal and has the same basic rights. Your goal is to learn to say 'no' in a calm, responsible manner without violating the rights of others. Being assertive is the desirable mid-path between being passive and aggressive.

Being too passive usually leads to loss of self-esteem and resentment. Learning how to effectively challenge the demands made on you by others is important if you are to deal with situations in a pleasant, relaxed manner, avoid misunderstandings and prevent yourself being persuaded to do things against your better judgement.

Learning to be assertive

Assertiveness skills are based on a few tried-and-tested techniques that give you the verbal tools to say 'no' politely and firmly. This helps you express your rights and can deal with many of the sources of stress in your life.

Basic assertion

This involves making a straightforward statement in which you calmly insist on your rights. Use a short statement that clearly sums up your needs, feelings or opinions. If, for example, your boss wants you to work on a Saturday, when you have made other plans, just say: 'I'm unable to work on Saturday.' When the person reinforces their argument, you do the same. 'I'm still unable to work on Saturday.' Never feel you have to explain – don't, for example, start telling your boss exactly what plans you have arranged for the weekend. This is irrelevant. Equally, don't feel you have to apologize – you have done nothing wrong!

The cracked record

This is a simple skill that is sometimes necessary when you need to be persistent in order to resist someone who is very persuasive. It merely depends on selecting a phrase and repeating it as often as necessary until the other person gives up trying to manipulate you. For example, just keep saying calmly, 'I am unable to work on Saturday at such short notice.' Keep repeating your statement each time the other person comes back with another demand or suggestion. If they don't respond after you have repeated your point, stay quiet – being comfortable with maintaining silence is vital since you need to state your case one more time than the other person makes their point.

Negotiation

It will usually help to reduce the tension if you can offer an acceptable compromise. 'No, I am unable to work this Saturday. However, I can work next Saturday and am willing to swap with anyone who can work this Saturday instead. Is that OK?' Keep calm and in control, and breathe slowly. Compromise makes everyone feel better as no one really loses. You have asserted your right not to change your plans at short notice, and have also offered your boss a possible solution to the dilemma.

Dealing with recurrent irritations

If someone repeatedly does something that upsets you, you need to deal with it calmly without causing resentment. It helps to work out a statement in advance that simply describes: the nature of the problem; how it affects you; how it makes you feel and how you would like it resolved.

If, for example, your boss keeps expecting you to work overtime on Saturdays, you could try to deal with it by saying: 'You keep expecting me to work overtime on Saturdays. This means I have little quality time with my family, which upsets me. I don't mind being flexible occasionally in an emergency, but I feel it is unreasonable to keep expecting me to work at the weekend. I would like to stick to my contracted hours more closely in future'.

Owning up

Asserting your rights also means taking responsibility for your own actions. If you make a mistake, it is important to acknowledge the fact. Say sorry, give your personal commitment that it will not happen again, and learn from the experience. This allows you to retain your self-respect and shows that you have sufficient confidence and maturity to take full responsibility for your behaviour. For example, if you agreed to do something by a certain time but failed, say, 'I apologize. I fully intended to complete this task by the agreed date, but it has taken longer than I expected. It is my fault and I will stay late tonight to ensure it is ready first thing tomorrow morning. This will not happen again.'

How to accept criticism

Being assertive and having more self-esteem means being able to accept constructive criticism but defending yourself against unearned criticism. For example, if someone says you are late, and you know this is true, agree by saying, 'Yes, I am sometimes late but I am trying to be more punctual.' If they unjustly say, 'You are always late,' and you are not, reply calmly: 'No, I am not always late. I have been late on only two occasions in the last three months.' Or you could ask for clarification. 'No, I am not always late at all. Why do you say that I am?'

Rational thinking

Rational thinking means overcoming common irrational ways of thinking, challenging upsetting thoughts, and thinking more positively. These skills will help you plan your thoughts rationally in a way that can help to lower your stress levels.

Psychologists have identified a number of common errors in the way people think when they are under pressure. These ways of thinking are essentially irrational and can significantly increase your stress levels. Try to avoid:

- FIXING LABELS such as 'I'm stupid', 'He's a loser', 'She's a complete idiot', 'I'm not good enough.'
- JUMPING TO CONCLUSIONS by mind-reading, such as, 'He must think I'm useless', 'They must think me stupid', 'She must be fed up with me by now'; or by fortune-telling, such as, 'I'm going to fail, I know I will', 'I know she won't like my work', 'There's no point in asking him, he's bound to refuse.'
- CONCENTRATING ON NEGATIVES AND IGNORING POSITIVES: 'Nothing's going right', 'Everyone hates me', 'I always mess up.'
- DOWNPLAYING POSITIVES: 'I only got invited because they needed some-one to make up the numbers', 'I only got that right through sheer luck', 'I only won that promotion because they need to keep me sweet.'
- THINKING IN ALL-OR-NOTHING TERMS: 'There's no point in trying as I'll never get it right', 'I have no option but to complain',

'I hate this, there's nothing good about it at all.'
- EXAGGERATING: 'That would be the worst thing ever to happen to me', 'If I don't do that, he'll kill me', 'If she ever finds out what happened, I'll die', 'I can't stand it any more.'
- ACCEPTING INAPPROPRIATE BLAME: 'The meeting went badly, it's all my fault', 'She didn't get that job – it's my fault for not coaching her properly', 'We failed to win that account – I'm to blame for giving a lousy presentation.'
- BLAMING OTHERS: 'It's all his fault – he should have warned me it was coming', 'It's all their fault for not thinking things through properly.'
- GENERALIZING: 'I always get it wrong', 'She's always late', 'Everyone's against me.'
- MINIMIZING EVENTS: 'I managed to pass, but it wasn't exactly with flying colours', 'He gave me a grade A, but I could have achieved an A-plus if I'd put more effort in.'
- LETTING YOUR EMOTIONS RULE: 'I feel stupid, so I must be', 'He made me feel upset, so he must be really horrible', 'I don't feel like doing that now, so I'll think about doing it later.'
- THINKING IN SHOULDS: 'I should have done that', 'He should have said so', 'I should try harder.'
- THINKING IN OUGHTS: 'I ought to say yes', 'I ought to do that', 'I ought to try harder.'
- THINKING IN MUSTS: 'I must do this', 'I must give in', 'I must say yes.'

Thinking more positively

It is common to compare yourself unfavourably with others, and this is a powerful source of internal stress. When you are under excess pressure, it helps to write down your thoughts and analyse them to see what errors you are making in the way you think. If you can eliminate these irrational thoughts, you will be able to deal with your stress more easily.

- If, for example, you are looking at a situation in black-and-white, all-or-nothing terms, or are exaggerating things, try to find some middle ground that helps you keep things in better perspective.

- If you find you are putting a label on someone as a result of their actions, is that label really justified?

- If you believe your own performance is poor, are you being too harsh on yourself? Where is the evidence? Try asking other people for their opinion and use their feedback in a positive, constructive manner to improve your performance where necessary, and to accept you've done well when you have.

- Don't make mountains out of molehills. It is common to use words that greatly exaggerate events. You may do this almost without thinking, and it can greatly increase the level of stress you feel in a particular situation. Look at the list of words opposite for suggestions on more realistic vocabulary.

Write down ten qualities you like about yourself (for example, sense of humour, good with children, patient, good cook, musical, interesting to talk to, caring, loyal, flexible). These are your ten aces – the things you like best about yourself, which no one can take away from you. Write this list of affirmations down again on a small piece of card, in order of their importance to you. Put this card in your wallet/purse and next time your self-esteem feels low or you feel you are not good enough, take that list out and read it. These are the top ten qualities that you like about yourself – and which others will appreciate and like, too. Feel free to add to the list until you have 20 or more qualities that make you feel good about yourself as a person. Read these as often as you need to boost your self-esteem.

Now write down ten qualities in yourself that you often feel negative about. You only feel bad about these qualities because you have somehow convinced yourself they are true. Isn't it surprising how easy it is to believe these negative thoughts and how difficult it is to believe the positive ones you wrote down in the previous exercise? The best thing to do with these negative thoughts is to turn them into positives. Go through the list of negatives, turn them into positives, and write these new positives down on another piece of card.

For example:

- 'I am not good enough' becomes 'I am good enough'
- 'I am not important' becomes 'I am as important as everyone else'
- 'I'm not very bright' becomes 'I am an intelligent human being'
- 'I'm not very interesting' becomes 'I am an interesting person'

- 'I'm not very lovable' becomes 'I am lovable'
- 'I don't really like myself' becomes 'I really like myself'
- 'I'm not very special' becomes 'I am special'
- 'I'm a nobody' becomes 'I am unique'
- 'I'm going nowhere' becomes 'I am capable of great things'
- 'It's too difficult' becomes 'I can do difficult things'
- 'I can't cope with change' becomes 'I can cope with change; changes are challenges and challenges are opportunities to learn'

Again, keep this list of adopted positive affirmations in your wallet/purse along with your other ten affirmations and refer to them whenever you start thinking negative thoughts about yourself. The more you read these affirmations, the more quickly they will become imprinted on your belief systems and the sooner they will start to improve your positive mental health.

Accepting criticism

Constructive criticism can be useful, but destructive criticism is something you want to offer up and forget about. It is not always easy to work out which is which at the time the criticism is made, however. You may need to go away and analyse what was said; whether the person was in a good mood or feeling vindictive, and whether or not they had your best interests at heart.

In the meantime, you need to know how to accept criticism so that you can see clearly whether it is constructive or destructive, and disarm the critic if necessary. It is important to stay relaxed, and to breathe slowly, deeply and calmly. Smile, lean slightly towards the person rather than drawing back, and don't respond until you've had time to think about what you want to say. The following techniques can help:

- First, pause and decide whether the criticism is valid: Yes? No? Maybe?

- If the criticism is valid:

    1. Agree with them: 'You're right, I can be untidy, but I'm working on it.'

    2. Thank them: 'Thank you for letting me know', or, 'That's a useful comment, I'll think about it/I'll take it on board', or, 'I'm glad you told me.'

    3. If necessary, apologize: 'I'm sorry. I'll take steps to put that right.'

    4. Learn from the criticism.

- If the criticism is invalid:

    1. Challenge them: 'Why are you saying that?'; 'Why do you feel the need to say that?'

    2. Ask for specifics: 'Would you mind telling me exactly what I did to make you say that?'

    3. Tell them you disagree with their assessment: 'I'm always willing to hear what you have to say. However, on this occasion I disagree for the following reasons…' If they continue to assert their criticism, say something along the lines of, 'Clearly we disagree. I still don't feel your criticism is valid.'

- If the criticism may be valid:

    1. Ask for clarification: 'Could you be more specific?' or, 'What exactly do you mean?'

    2. Ask their advice: 'How would you have done that differently?'

- If they were unkind enough to make the criticism in front of someone else, you could draw the other person in if you are sure you are on firm ground: 'What do you think?' or, 'Do you agree?' or, 'Do you believe that's the case?'

Consider criticism a gift – an opportunity to improve if the criticism is valid, and an opportunity to re-affirm your self-esteem if the criticism is invalid. Put-downs can only really hurt you if you believe there is a nugget of truth in what is being said. If, for example, someone criticized you by saying, 'You have green hair', this would not hurt at all and you would easily laugh it off. If, however, they said, 'You're lazy', this would hurt if you secretly thought it might be true. If you know you are not lazy, but the criticism has still hurt, add 'I am not lazy' to the list of affirmations in your wallet/purse.

Improving relationships

Good communication is important in all relationships, whether they involve your parents, children, friends, colleagues, boss, acquaintances or anyone else you need to deal with. Good communication means:

- Expressing yourself clearly and assertively: say what you mean, and mean what you say. Don't use veiled hints and comments.

- Listening carefully to others: both to hear what they are saying, and to check how well you have been understood.

- Reaching an agreed endpoint where you both know what is happening and how things will progress, if necessary.

Expressing yourself

Expressing yourself properly means exploring your feelings in order to understand exactly how you feel about a particular situation; recognizing that certain issues need to be dealt with rather than passively endured; and acting assertively to protect your rights.

- To express yourself well, you need to choose the right time and place for making your statement. Some issues need to be dealt with immediately. Other, more long-term problems should be addressed in private when you both have time to deal with the problem fully.

- Choose a phrase that succinctly sums up what you want to say. Use 'I' language: 'I feel', 'I would prefer', 'I would like'. Rather than 'you' language: 'You must', 'You should', and so on.

- Stick to the point without nagging or getting sidetracked.

- If you are dealing with a problem that annoys or upsets you, use a formula that states what the problem is (for example, 'You were late again this morning'); how this affects you (for example, 'I was left hanging around for half an hour'); how this makes you feel (for example, 'I felt annoyed and upset'); how you would like the issue resolved (for example, 'Please make sure you do not leave me waiting again') – this is the desirable endpoint that you are requesting.

- Listen to their response to ensure they have understood what you have said, have taken it on board, and agree. If they do not agree, then you may have to agree to differ.

If the tables are turned, and you are the one being criticized, tips on the best way to deal with this are given on page 204.

Learning to listen

Being a good listener is a skill that others will quickly appreciate.

- Using plenty of eye contact, give verbal encouragement: use words such as 'Uh-huh?', 'Really?'

- Give non-verbal encouragement: nod your head, or animate your face to reflect what you are hearing – look sad, happy, interested, amused or concerned as appropriate.

- Don't interrupt until the person has had their say. Don't be tempted to finish their sentence for them.

- Reply appropriately with a phrase that sums up what you have heard.

- Make a suitable closing statement: 'Let's go and have a cup of tea while you try to relax and calm down.' Or, 'That was a great story, but we'd better get back to work now.' This is the desirable endpoint you are suggesting, or that the other person is requesting.

Developing hobbies and interests

A well-rounded, self-confident person is aware of the world around them, keeps up-to-date with current affairs and develops a number of hobbies and areas of special interest. These interests are what help to define you as an individual and what helps to make your conversation stimulating and educational. Hobbies that involve joining groups or taking classes are also an excellent way of meeting like-minded people with whom you are likely to have a lot in common.

It is important to have at least one hobby or interest outside your work and family life. Hobbies can help you keep fit (for example, gardening, DIY, swimming, golf, bowling, tennis, rambling, jogging, dancing); they can exercise your mind (for example, doing crosswords, studying for an exam, teaching yourself chess or Egyptian hieroglyphics); and can even provide extra income (for example, creative writing, buying and selling antiques or stamps). Hobbies can also be spiritually rewarding (for example, bird-watching, voluntary work, visiting the elderly and lonely).

List the hobbies that you indulge in and list the activities you have often thought about doing but never got around to. Promise yourself that you will start at least one of these activities within the next two weeks.

7 STREAMLINE YOUR LIFE

And finally, to help ensure that high stress levels remain a thing of the past, the last step in this seven-point plan looks at practical ways to keep life running as smoothly as possible.

Making time for relaxation

Whether you work at home, away from home or in the home it is helpful to streamline certain aspects of your domestic life to help free up more time for rest and relaxation.

Organizational skills are as useful in the home as they are at work. Delegate jobs to others where appropriate and ensure that you are not put upon to do more than your fair share of chores.

It will help to set a routine as much as possible. This is especially important if there are times of the day when you tend to function less efficiently, such as early morning or late evening. Before going to bed, for example, do whatever you can to minimize tomorrow's morning rush, such as laying the breakfast table and getting out the clothes you intend to wear. Always eat breakfast, even if up until now you haven't made time. Breakfast is the most important meal of the day when you are under pressure (see Chapter 3).

An excellent tip to help save time is to get up when you wake up rather than lying in bed. You could even set your alarm clock an hour earlier than usual and get up to go for a gentle jog or even a swim to get you off to a good start for the day. It is often more pleasant to exercise when you are feeling fresh rather than at the end of a long, tiring day.

Being organized means doing jobs when they need doing rather than putting them off until they have to be done. Rather than transferring dirty clothes from the bedroom laundry basket into the 'waiting-to-be-washed' basket in the utility room, put them straight into the washing machine and set the machine going.

Self-help

- Keep pen and paper (or if you prefer, a dictaphone) by your bed so you can write down important thoughts that come into your head while going to sleep.

- Write Post-It notes to yourself to remind yourself to do things and stick them somewhere obvious where you will see them, such as on the fridge door, or on the kitchen table. Discard them when they have fulfilled their purpose.

- Assign a usual place for important items (for example, keys) and do your best to ensure they are always returned there after use.

- Limit your wardrobe of clothes, and their colours, so you spend less time thinking about what to wear. This is especially easy for clothes you wear around the house (for example, leggings, T-shirt, cardigan).

- Eliminate jobs around the house that aren't essential – it isn't usually necessary to vacuum every day, for example.

- Delegate as many jobs to others as you can afford (for example, invest in a domestic help to vacuum, dust and iron; a gardener to mow your lawn; a friendly teenager to wash your car).

- Assign chores (for example, putting out the bins, loading the dishwasher) to other family members – use a rota if necessary.

- Keep a selection of greetings cards at home so you always have a suitable last-minute card available for a birthday or celebration.

- Whenever you buy something new, try to get rid of something old.

- Keep financial papers, bills, insurance, mortgage details, birth certificates, wills, etc. all together in one lockable desk or file box.

- Use direct debit facilities to pay as many bills as possible.

- Make a list of things that really matter to you and spend more time doing these – and less time on everything else.

- Spend at least 20 minutes relaxing in the evening before going to bed. Indulge in an aromatherapy bath and review your day in your mind as well as thinking about things you would like to do tomorrow.

Goal planning

Goal planning is important in all aspects of your life, for you can only achieve your goals if you know exactly what they are. Spend a little time thinking realistically about where you would like to be in one year's time, five years' time and then ten years' time.

Your goals should encompass all areas of your life, including your personal life, career, financial standing, work-related skills, qualifications, experiences, abilities and qualities. Set realistic short- and long-term goals that do not conflict with one another. If you want to spend more time studying, for example, it may be difficult to spend more quality time with your partner, too. Don't pile too much pressure on yourself, as unrealistic goals can be a source of stress in themselves, and multiple failures to achieve those goals will also erode your self-esteem.

Once you have written down your lists, keep them somewhere safe such as in your wallet or purse, where you can refer to them regularly to keep them firmly fixed in your mind.

Now consider where you are now in relation to where you want to be. You then need to draw up a plan that will help you to achieve your goals and you will then need to hold regular self-audit sessions to see how far along the road you are. Only by honestly assessing your progress and by reformulating or reinforcing your goals are you likely get to where you want to be.

Controlling perfectionism

No one is perfect, yet many people waste a lot of time trying to be so. Perfectionism involves getting everything exactly right, down to the last detail. This is usually a waste of precious time, however, because, according to the Law of Diminishing Returns, the more time you spend on the minutiae of a particular task, the less you will achieve per unit of time. Even worse than wasting time is the very real risk that not getting something right will be deemed as a failure by your hardest task-master – you. Even if they get something 99 per cent right, a perfectionist will focus only on the 1 per cent of the task that was wrong.

Getting something wrong can be an advantage, however, as it means you then have an opportunity to learn from your mistakes. Everyone is allowed to make mistakes and you should be comfortable with that. Otherwise, you may subconsciously start to fear making mistakes and avoid undertaking new challenges because of your fear of failure.

- Set yourself a time-limit for a particular task.

- If at the end of this time, the task is still not completed to your satis-faction, allow yourself an additional short deadline and no more.

- Adopt the saying, 'It is better to have tried and failed, than not to have tried at all.'

- Make sure that all the resources you need are available before starting a task – and warn others if necessary that you may well fail at a par-ticular task but you are still willing to give it your best shot.

Time management

Time is a finite commodity – a fact that is easy to forget when you are stressed and working long hours. The best way to remember the importance of time management is to consider this equation:

Quality Time (leisure, family, sport)

+ **Work Time** (getting to and from the workplace, paper-pushing, telephoning, planning, finances, feeling stressed)

= **Total Time** (i.e., the sum total of your adult life)

The more time you spend on work and feeling stressed, the less time is available for rest, relaxation, recuperation and fun. Your battle cry should be that you work to live, not that you live to work, and it is important to make work time as efficient as possible to prevent it eating into quality time.

Manage time firmly or it will happily manage you. The most important skills of time management are prioritizing tasks and delegation.

Prioritizing

When managing time, it is vital to do the most important and pressing jobs first before turning your attention to those that can wait a little longer.

Making a 'To Do' list

A 'To Do' list will help you improve your organizational skills and prioritize tasks so that the most important get done first. You can buy printed tear-off booklets designed for such lists or you can draw up your own.

1. Make a list of all the tasks you need to do during the next few days.

2. Put them in order of importance using an A, B, C coding, for example, A1, A2, A3. Jobs labelled A are urgent, Bs are less immediate but should not be left too long. Cs are non-urgent but still represent important tasks.

3. Add to the list during the day as new tasks appear, and tick off items as they are completed.

4. At the end of each day, rewrite your list, re-prioritizing the coding as necessary.

As you review your list you will notice that some items follow a regular pattern – they stay static, appear often or move up and down.

- If they remain static, can you justify having them on your list? *Do* them, or remove them as unimportant.

- If an item appears regularly, consider whether you can remove it by delegating the task to someone else.

- If the item moves up and down but doesn't get done, consider why. Are you dithering or avoiding the issue?

Delegating

Delegation is the art of freeing up your own time and resources by donating a task previously under your control to someone else who is equally capable of performing it. Some people find delegation easy, while others find it hard. In some cases, giving up a job may mean shedding a boring or onerous task, but it also means giving up some control and admitting to yourself that you are not indispensable for this particular task. People with good self-esteem are usually good delegators, while those with poor self-esteem may find it difficult to hand over responsibilities to others.

A job cannot be done properly if no one knows what the job entails, however, so communication is important when delegating important tasks. Those who know what is expected of them and who are given incentives to achieve it tend to be the most loyal and hard-working. It may help to:

- Write down exactly what is expected of the person to whom you are delegating a complex task.

- Hold a regular forum for communication. Allow feedback. Give praise when it's due. Reprimand fairly and *not* in public.

- Give an incentive for peole to meet an important goal.

- Learn to give authority yet at the same time retain responsibility.

RESOURCES

Please send a large, stamped, self-addressed envelope when writing to the following addresses.

Alcohol

Alcohol Concern
Waterbridge House
32-36 Loman St
London SE1 0EE
(020 7928 7377)
www.alcoholconcern.org.uk
Information service.

Drinkline
(0800 917 8282)
National alcohol helpline.

Alternative therapies

British Herbal Medicine Association
Sun House
Church St
Stroud GL5 1JL
(01453 751389)
www.bhma.info
Information leaflets, booklets,
compendium, telephone advice.

British Homeopathic Association
15 Clerkenwell Close
London EC1R 0AA
(020 7566 7800)
Send SAE for list of medically qualified
homeopathic doctors.

British Reflexology Association
Monks Orchard
Whitbourne
Worcester WR6 5RB
(01886 821 207)
www.britreflex.co.uk

General Council and Register of Naturopaths
Goswell House
2 Goswell Road
Street
Somerset
BA 16 0JG
(08707 456984)
www.naturopathy.org.uk

Massage Therapy Institute of Great Britain
PO Box 2726
London NW2 3NR
(020 7724 7198)

The Register of Chinese Herbal Medicine
Office 5, Ferndale Business Centre
1 Exeter Street
Norwich NR2 4QB
(01603 623 994)
www.rchm.co.uk
Send an SAE and £3.00.

Anxiety/stress

International Stress Management Association
PO Box 348
Waltham Cross
EN8 8ZL
(07000 780430)
www.isma.org.uk

Bereavement

CRUSE – Bereavement Care
Cruse House
126 Sheen Road
Richmond
Surrey TW9 1UR
(020 8939 9530)
(0870 1671677 (helpline))
www.crusebereavementcare.org.uk
Offers counselling, advice and social contacts for all bereaved people.

Counselling

British Association for Behavioural and Cognitive Psychotherapy
BABCP General Office
Globe Centre
PO Box 9
Accrington BB5 2GD
(01254 875277)
www.babcp.org.uk

British Association for Counselling
1 Regent Place
Rugby Warwickshire CV21 2PJ
(0870 4435252)
www.bac.co.uk
Send an SAE for a register of local accredited counsellors and a publication list.

British Confederation of Psychotherapists
37 Mapesbury Road
London NW2 4HJ
(020 8830 5173)
www.bcp.org.uk
Provides a register of psychotherapists and a free brochure, 'Finding a Therapist'.

Depression

Depression Alliance
35 Westminster Bridge Road
London SE1 7JB
(020 7633 0557)
www.depressionalliance.org

Samaritans
(08457 909090)
www.samaritans.org.uk

Hair Loss

Attention X
316 King Street
Hammersmith
London W6 0RR
(020 8741 8224)
Medical hair design to disguise trichotillomania and alopecia, etc.

Herbal suppliers

The Nutri-Centre
The Hale Clinic
7 Park Crescent
London WIB 1PF
(020 7436 5122)
www.nutricentre.com
Supplies many of the aromatherapy,

herbal and homeopathic supplements mentioned in this book by mail order.

Impotence

Impotence Association
PO Box 10296
London SW17 9WH
(confidential helpline: 020 8767 7791, 9am–5pm)
www.impotence.org.uk
Please send a large stamped SAE for the leaflet 'Impotence Explained – A Couples' Guide to Erectile Dysfunction'.

Premenstrual syndrome

National Association for Premenstrual Syndrome
41 Old Road
East Peckham
TN12 5AP
(0870 777 2177)
www.pms.org.uk

Premenstrual Society
PO Box 429
Addlestone
Surrey KT15 1DZ
(01932 872 560)

Relationship problems

Relate
Herbert Gray College
Little Church Street
Rugby
Warwickshire CV21 3AP
(01788 573241)
www.relate.org.uk
Works to support marriage and family life by providing counselling and sex therapy for couples with relationship problems at more than 120 local centres nationwide.

Smoking

QUIT
102 Gloucester Place
London W1H 3DA
(Quitline 0800 00 2200)
Advice and counselling on giving up smoking.

INDEX